Science & Practice of

Integrative Health & Wellbeing Lifestyle

Science & Practice of Integrative Health & Wellbeing Lifestyle

A handbook for everyone to explore and embrace an Integrated Lifestyle informed by Modern Medicine, Ayurveda, Yoga, and Meditation

Krishnamurthy Jayanna

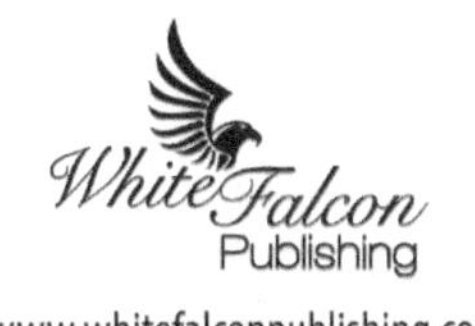

White Falcon Publishing

www.whitefalconpublishing.com

Science & Practice of Integrative Health & Wellbeing Lifestyle
Krishnamurthy Jayanna

www.whitefalconpublishing.com

INSPIRATION

Dr. Kamlesh D. Patel, fondly referred to as Daaji, has been an inspiring force behind this book and the work that it represents. He is the Global Guide of Heartfulness practice and is guiding millions of seekers all over the world in adopting Heart based meditation and embracing the Heartful Way of Life. Daaji refers to himself as a student of spirituality, while being a Master and an adept in the field of Meditation and Yoga. He is a keen observer and a researcher himself, a strong advocate of integrating the best of modern and traditional science of wellbeing.

Heartfulness Institute is a non-profit organization providing training and support to the interested seekers and institutions in more than 160 countries through its team of volunteers. These services are offered free of charge as policy and principle followed, right from the inception of this practice, more than a century ago. The organization has various formats and customized trainings and tools for communities and institutions from all backgrounds: corporates, universities, schools, health, and hospitality sector, etc. Most recently, the organization has responded to the Covid-19 pandemic through donations, food, and other support services to the needy, counseling, and meditation support through helplines. Revenues out of this book will serve the noble vision of this organization.

DEDICATION

To all those on the path of Lifestyle Change

as Explorers,

as Advocates and,

as Champions.

LOVING MEMORY

Our dear mother, Mangala Jayanna who breathed her last due to cancer, last year. She was the champion of an ideal lifestyle in many ways: she woke up early, meditated at a fixed hour, regularly walked and did yoga, chose foods consciously, slept early, and she did all this naturally and joyfully. And we saw how her integrative lifestyle enriched her quality of life throughout her lifetime. Her endurance to go through the final stages of cancer in peace and acceptance showed us how meditation had impacted her inner wellbeing and supported her from the inside while complementing the best efforts of modern medicine from the outside.

Her subtle presence and thoughts surround us and continue to inspire us. She demonstrated to us how an integrative lifestyle can prepare us for all the stages of life.

PREFACE

The year 2020 is significant in the field of global public health. The world is witnessing the global pandemic due to a novel Corona Virus, named as Covid-19. What started as an outbreak in Wuhan, China, in November- December 2019 has quickly spread to more than 200 countries infecting over 33 million people and killing close to 1,000,000 individuals in just about ten months. Developed nations that had the highest standards of public health and clinical infrastructure, such as the USA, Italy, Spain have not been spared. For a country like India, with its 1.3 billion population, the problem presents itself as a unique public health crisis.

The pandemic and the lockdown have given our world its much-needed pause and has forced us to face some hard questions. One that is of paramount importance is the lifestyle, which not only results in outbreaks such as this but also facilitates rapid transmission affecting millions. This is happening too frequently these years. Ebola outbreak and the SARS are still fresh in our minds. Did we not expect this? Why weren't we prepared? Could we have done something to prevent this? While protective measures and vaccines have been discussed and will continue to be discussed, a more fundamental question arises: *Are they enough?*

Even as we develop new vaccines, will the viruses not mutate, and will there not be other viruses? *Should we look at these challenges at a more fundamental level?*

Are the human practices and lifestyles that give rise to these outbreaks not important to address?

Are there lifestyle interventions, behaviors, practices that can strengthen immunity in a more fundamental way? Is this not an important research question to pursue?

We can list a good number of lifestyle attributes that facilitate the occurrence and rapid transmission of these outbreaks: human-animal contact, food practices, travel, personal hygiene, working conditions, physical and mental wellbeing, etc.

For a second, let us forget the Corona outbreak. The other conditions, such as diabetes, cardiovascular diseases, mental health, and cancers also have an association with lifestyle changes. The statistics related to these conditions are staggering. More than 40 million deaths every year are due to non-communicable diseases, and this group alone constitutes 71% of all deaths globally. Of these numbers, the break up is as follows: cardiovascular diseases (18 million), diabetes (1.6 million), respiratory diseases (3.9 million), and cancers (9 million) and others. 15 million of the 40 million deaths occur in the age group of 30 to 69 years and are referred to as premature deaths. WHO lists rapid unplanned urbanization, globalization of unhealthy lifestyles, and population aging as the forces driving these deaths.

How do we fix this? This calls for action individually and collectively.

This book is primarily intended to serve as a handbook or a practical guide to help the reader get a glimpse of the lifestyle issues that we face today and plan some practical steps toward changing them.

Prevention and health promotion through lifestyle modification is rightly the focus of integrated health and wellbeing lifestyle. We particularly advocate for the integration of modern with traditional disciplines such as Ayurveda, Yoga, and Meditation. There has been growing interest and research in these disciplines and their effects on health and wellbeing; they have the potential to complement well with modern medicine and can seamlessly integrate into one's lifestyle.

While this lockdown is not without its inconveniences, it has provided time and space for serious reflection and course correction. It is our hope that this book provides the reader with useful and practical guidance as well as inspiration to relook at ones lifestyle through a new lens.

Krishnamurthy Jayanna

ABOUT THE HANDBOOK

What is this handbook about?

This book is intended to be a simple, user-friendly, and practical guide to adopt an integrative lifestyle for enhancing the quality of life.

Who is this handbook for?

This book is meant for everyone, from all age groups and backgrounds: women and children, working professionals, middle-aged and elderly, anyone who is keen on continuous improvement of one's lifestyle.

This book provides insights to professionals who are interested in studying or providing integrative health and wellbeing services.

Why is this called a handbook?

The purpose of this book is to provide simple and practical guidance to the reader, at a pace that is decided by the reader. The book has information synthesized out of the latest scientific evidence in the field of Lifestyle Medicine as well as science and philosophy of ancient disciplines such as Ayurveda, Yoga, and Meditation. Our intent is to have this compilation available as a handy tool at all times during the day and year as a continuous resource to facilitate a lifestyle change.

Who is behind this handbook?

We are a team of people from multiple disciplines and backgrounds that come together under the umbrella of "Center for Integrative Health and Wellbeing" or "CIHW". CIHW has two pillars: Health and Education. ANIRASA is the clinical pillar of CIHW that provides integrative lifestyle services. Our team members comprise of Ayurveda physicians, Yoga instructors, Meditation trainers, Researchers, Public Health professionals, Educationists, and Technologists. Our vision is to educate and support individuals, families, and institutions in embracing a lifestyle that blends the science and philosophy of modern and traditional sciences of healing.

ORGANIZATION OF THE HANDBOOK

The handbook is organized into five broad sections.

Introduction: Background Theory (BT) Series

Here we present some theoretical knowledge that is synthesized from standard texts and scientific articles and forms the basis of lifestyle that we advocate as Integrative Health and Wellbeing Lifestyle.

Preparing for Lifestyle Change: Good to Know (GtK) Series

This section has some facts that are good to know, interesting, and can motivate us for a change. It is presented in a simple style for easy assimilation and adoption; there are 22 chapters within the four disciplines: Lifestyle Medicine, Ayurveda, Yoga, and Meditation.

Making Lifestyle Change: Inspired Action (IA) Series

Knowledge alone is not enough to sustain behavior change. There are more fundamental forces, inspiring one toward sustainable change, discussed in this section. Five chapters are dedicated to this section.

Lifestyle Change for Common Conditions: Practical Integrated Approach (PIA) Series

Integrative approaches to a few common conditions are presented in this section. The intention is not to provide any new protocol or treatment as there are good protocols that already exist. The idea is to draw focus on the integrative lifestyle changes specific to the disease conditions. Five chapters come under this section, Practical Integrative Approach (PIA).

Resources Tools and Support (RTS)

This section provides annexures related to tools, references, and other resources that support practical application and adoption of lifestyle practices.

HOW TO APPROACH
THIS BOOK?

This book is primarily intended to be a handbook or a practical guide to assist you in gaining some awareness and plan your actions. This is not a detailed reference book nor a textbook that provides a sequence of events in a particular direction.

So, you can essentially pick up any section or chapter and start reading it. Each section or chapter is discrete in itself and provides you with some input.

Each chapter is intentionally developed as a small article ranging from 2 to 4 pages, and it will help if you can take up one chapter at a time and read it thoroughly.

Probably one chapter per day is a great start. We advise you to maintain a journal or a diary by your side.

After you read a chapter, you may highlight those words or lines that appealed to you most.

Reflect over them and write down the additional insights that you gain and the action points that you are inspired to plan in your journal.

You may also want to do more research in those areas and start adding your knowledge base in that area. Some references are provided in the end, and they can be a good start.

Are you someone who would like to know the roots first, of the philosophy and the science? Then, 'Background Theory' can be a good start.

Are you someone who would like to quickly dive into the practical aspect? The Good to Know section will provide some theory and simple practical guidance to start changing one's lifestyle.

Do you directly want to jump into the specific conditions? You are free to take a dive.

It is your handbook, your personal guide, and you are the driver.

All the best.

Feel free to write to us for any clarifications, comments, and suggestions. You can reach us at cihw@cihw.in

ACKNOWLEDGMENTS

Many have contributed to this book, directly and indirectly.

Foremost, my wife Ramya has been a strong supporter of this initiative from the time of inception and leads many aspects of the center. For the book, she supported in various ways: design, content simplification, content editing, and content organization.

Our clinical team: Dr. Suchetha Sarathy and Dr. Smitha, Ayurveda physicians; Mrs. Jayanthi Subranyam, Yoga instructor; Mrs. Usha Amol, Meditation trainer and clinic coordinator; Mrs. Shobha Amarnath, who leads the education vertical of the center; Mr. Manjunatha G. M., partner on the ANIRASA clinic initiative, have supported in many ways through knowledge sharing, ideas, perspectives and motivation which have led to this book.

We acknowledge the following who continue to support the center's activities in many ways: Ms. Jeevitha Ramesh, Ms. Sandhya Basu, Dr. Shashi Kumar, Dr. Manjunatha R., Dr. Sunil S., Dr. Sriharsha M. L., Dr. Kiran Rao, and some who were with us in the initial part of the journey: Madhavi B., Dr. Swathi N. and Ms. Sreenidhi S.

At the home front, our father, K. N. Jayanna, and our two sons Ramesh and Nikhil; my brother, Mohan Kumar have been a strong support and backbone in all that we do. We also remember and thank the rest of our family members, friends, well-wishers, and colleagues who continue to encourage us.

Our gratitude to all our brothers and sisters of the Heartfulness family who are a source of constant support and inspiration behind this work.

Heartfulness Institute gave permission to use the information about Heartfulness practices in the annexures. Several images and information were referenced from various articles and websites that are duly cited.
xxii

Disclaimer: The views expressed in this book are solely of the author and do not represent the official policy or position of the institutions that he is affiliated to.

CONTENTS

SECTION 4
Lifestyle Change for Common Conditions:
Practical Integrative Approach (PIA) Series

SECTION 5
Annexures: *Resources, Tools, and Support*

SECTION 1

Introduction:
Background Theory (BT) Series

1 BT 1: Health, Wellbeing, and Quality of Life: *Changing Paradigm*

*I*n this chapter, we will explore the ideas and concepts of health, wellbeing, and quality of life and how our current lifestyles are affecting them.

Let us first explore the current global health agenda.

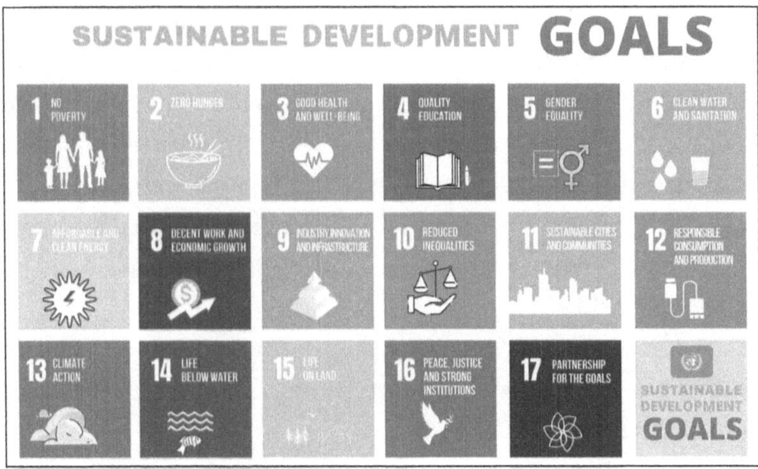

Sustainable Development Goals (SDGs) are a set of global goals related to major challenges concerning the development of humanity and the ecosystem today. They are 17 in number concerning various facets of development, and the third goal (SDG 3) refers to 'Health and Wellbeing'. The goal encourages every country to ensure healthy lives and promote wellbeing for all at all ages by 2030.

Compared to the previous set of goals, called Millennium Development Goals (MDG) that were the focus between 1990 and 2015, the SDGs are more in number (17 compared to 8) and have a wider focus. While MDG health goals focused mostly on saving lives, SDGs bring a stronger focus on wellbeing in addition to saving lives.

And, this has come at a time when the health pattern across the world is going through a major transition.

In the early 1900s, the average life expectancy globally was 30 years of age, i.e., the majority of the people lived only up to 30 years, and people died mostly due to infectious (communicable) diseases such as malaria, measles, and polio. With the progress in vaccines, diagnostics, antibiotics, specialization of care, and public health infrastructure, life expectancy has increased to over 71 years today. Now the common causes of deaths are non-communicable diseases such as cardiovascular diseases, cancers, and diabetes. These are also referred to as lifestyle diseases as they are the result of changes in living conditions and lifestyle of people in the modern world.

Although people are living longer, they are not necessarily healthier as non-communicable diseases are chronic in nature and lifelong.

Despite great strides and ever-increasing investments in medical infrastructure, diagnostics, specialization, drug discovery, and other treatment modalities, most of these diseases remain non-curable. At best, they can be controlled. Additionally, we also observe an increase in mental health conditions such as depression, stress, and anxiety and neurological disorders such as Alzheimer's and Parkinsonism, all that significantly affect the wellbeing and quality of life of not only the patients but also the families. So, bringing the focus on wellbeing within the SDGs is indeed a welcome change.

Now, let us dive deeper into the ideas and concepts of health, wellbeing, and quality of life.

WHO defined 'Health' as a 'state of complete physical, mental, and social wellbeing and not merely the absence of disease or infirmity'.

This definition was found to be very relevant in the post-world war scenario when life expectancy was lower, and most deaths were due to infectious diseases. There is a growing feeling and criticism in recent years that this definition is outdated and not applicable in today's context of disease pattern. Researchers and activists have expressed that this definition is very idealistic and not practical; it will continue to attract huge investments and resources for something that is not practically feasible.

With the change of times and change of disease pattern, should the definition be revisited?

Or, should it continue to provide a vision of high order to inspire everyone: the provider, the client, and other stakeholders to aim for the highest? These questions will continue to be debated for a long time.

Every disease has an objective dimension that is visible to the physician, and also a subjective dimension that the patient experiences, but may not be visible externally. The positive subjective experience of wellbeing is referred to as wellness, and the negative experience as illness, which often may go unnoticed due to various reasons. A growing body of evidence is shedding light on how wellbeing and quality of life have been impacted by chronic diseases, but since they are not visible, they do not get sufficient attention.

What are these subjective notions of wellbeing and quality of life?

Wellbeing includes subjective and psychological dimensions which are derived from Hedonic and Eudemonic ideas of happiness, in Greek philosophy; Hedonic refers to pleasure derived directly out of external things, and Eudemonic refers to pleasure derived out of the meaning of things, the latter leading to personal (inner) fulfillment.

The subjective wellbeing includes measures such as life satisfaction (personal happiness), presence or absence of disease (positive and negative affect). The psychological wellbeing measures functional dimensions such as autonomy, personal growth, self-acceptance, purpose in life, environmental mastery, and positive relations with others.

Wellness, in another context, is defined as a holistic integration of physical, mental, and spiritual wellbeing, fueling the body, engaging the mind, and nurturing the spirit. Eight dimensions of wellness are provided.

Quality of life has also attracted much attention in recent years. It includes many dimensions of wellbeing in it.

WHO defines Quality of Life as "individuals' perception of their position in life in the context of the culture and value systems in which they live and in relation to their goals, expectations, standards, and concerns".

As we dive deeper into these ideas, one gets the sense of how complex and subjective they are; and challenging to address in a given hospital or a clinic setting. Yet, it is the need of the hour as we observe that wellbeing and quality of life are declining globally.

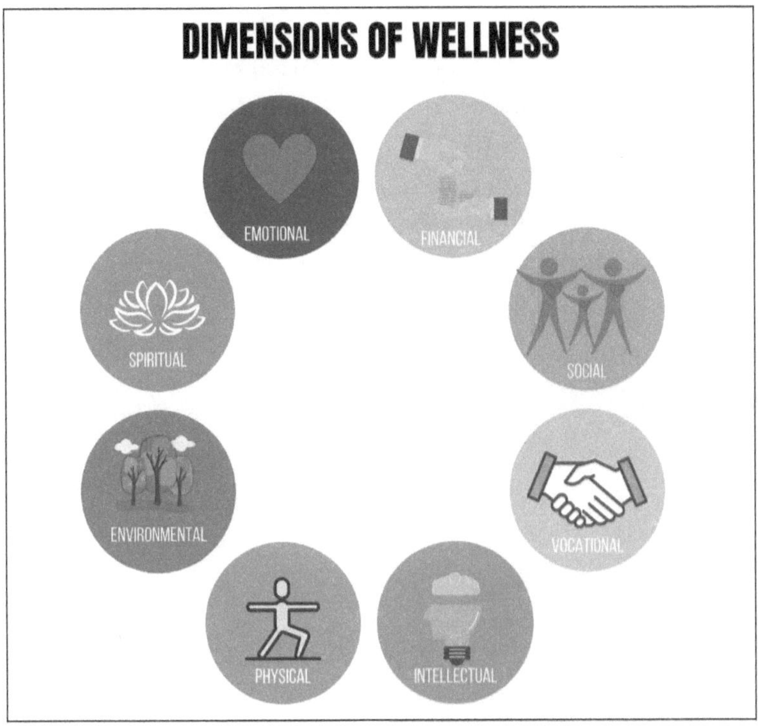

Strong evidence suggests that it is the changing lifestyles that are impacting wellbeing and quality of life.

We are quite aware as to what has led to the change in our lifestyles: globalization and urbanization, changing living conditions, social and family systems, work culture, travel, changing food practices, etc. In this backdrop, lifestyle change needs attention while considering social and cultural contexts.

While non-communicable diseases dominate the picture today, communicable diseases continue to attract attention too.

Severe Acute Respiratory Syndrome (SARS), Middle East Respiratory Syndrome (MERS), Ebola virus outbreak, and the most recent, novel Corona Virus disease (Covid-19) are related to many behavioral and lifestyle aspects that characterize today's world. In the modern globalized world, an outbreak in one part of the world can quickly assume pandemic proportions killing a few million in a short time.

So, lifestyles assume greater importance today than ever before. Many attempts have been made to address them. Let us explore what progress we have made in this area in the subsequent chapters.

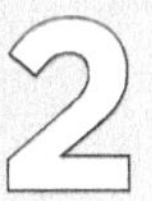

BT 2: Lifestyle Interventions and Challenges: *Unanswered Questions*

In the previous chapter, we discussed the current status of health and wellbeing and the need to address them through lifestyle interventions. In this chapter, we will explore the challenges and practical considerations in implementing them.

While there is a general understanding that wellbeing and quality of life are important and need to be addressed, they are not simple. Their subjective dimensions extend beyond the scope of the conventional health domain.

Let us take the ideas of personal happiness or self-acceptance in the context of someone just diagnosed with cancer. The health sector can do everything possible with diagnosis and managing cancer to save the life of the patient. The subjective ideas of happiness and acceptance of the patient often enter into religious and personal spiritual spaces. There are also socio-cultural aspects and the role of the patient as well as the family that needs to be taken into account.

It is practically impossible for a physician or a nurse or even a counselor working within a hospital or a clinic to address the wide range of complex issues that surround the wellbeing and quality of life.

Time is a constrained resource in hospitals that have long waiting lines of patients. Training and competency are yet another set of gaps to address these complex and subjective issues.

Imagine a case of terminal cancer when the best of the standard therapeutics are failing, and the client and the family are deeply emotional and low in morale. Or take an example of a chronic diabetic in whom blood sugar levels continue to fluctuate, despite taking medication and complying with visits and check-ups. In either case, what is going on in the deeper subjective realms of mind or the body or how the other stressors are affecting the psychology or the physiology, is hard to understand and address.

Here arises the relevance of some of the traditional healing methods such as Meditation, Yoga, Tai-chi, Ayurveda, and others.

There is a growing body of literature on how these interventions can impact health, wellbeing, and quality of life and that they can complement modern medicine in several ways. This will be dealt with in greater detail in the subsequent chapters.

There is also a need to address lifestyles at various stages: before the onset of disease as part of prevention, as part of general health promotion, during disease management after the onset of disease, and also in the end stages when the disease is no more manageable. Quality of life takes precedence at all stages, and our health systems need to be equipped with multidisciplinary capacities.

However, how best can other disciplines be integrated within the mainstream service delivery is an area that is not explored as much.

Within conventional or modern medicine, there is a tendency to focus on a specific intervention or a drug or a vaccine. In contrast, something like a lifestyle and behavior change is perceived as complex and hard to deliver. Multiple disciplines coming together and working in harmony with a focus on the client demands attention by both the policy leaders and the providers in the frontline. Health systems tend to lean toward curing and managing diseases as that has been the focus all along, and there is a need to think very differently within the systems to bring the focus onto disease prevention or lifestyle change.

Clients too have challenges in managing their current living conditions that do not allow them to prioritize preventive lifestyles. This is true for individuals from all socio-economic strata.

Think of a daily wage earner who has relocated to an urban area from a village in rural India. He or she may not be too motivated to prioritize a lifestyle change that will prevent disease occurrence in the future. Tomorrow is simply too distant for them. Similarly, a global consultant who is traveling a few months in a year and is on a continuous pressure to meet deadlines may find it hard to bring about the desired level of the lifestyle change that is ideal.

Thus, there is a need to address it at both ends: providers and clients.

This approach enters into the realm of public health to address the demand and supply-side perspectives; study the convergence of different disciplines while addressing the socio-cultural-demographics surrounding the issue. This should translate into simple tools and interventions for individuals both from upper and lower socioeconomic strata to manage lifestyle change in a practical way. Operations and implementation research is the need of the hour to study the convergence and integrated delivery of these interventions. Few questions arise in this regard:

How do we equip our health infrastructure to integrate health and wellbeing services in a way that is effective and simple for providers to deliver, and for the clients to participate and benefit?

How do we motivate the behaviors of the people at large, to be able to prioritize prevention and lifestyle change while still being healthy?

How do we achieve these changes at a level that produces a population-wide impact?

It becomes a priority for the global and national health policies to research some of these questions and explore solutions, in the years to come, to make the SDG aspirations a reality.

The Government of India has begun its exploration in this space through its new program – Ayushman Bharat, where there is an attempt to provide preventive and health promotion services through the health and wellness centers all across the country. This is a good beginning, but many practical and operational hurdles are still to be crossed. The scope of the intervention package is still limited. Some of the client-specific subjective issues of wellbeing and quality of life that we discussed will require a new lens to explore.

Integrative Health and Wellbeing lifestyle is an idea that is still new and will demand certain rigor and investment into infrastructure, research, and training in the future.

Subsequent chapters in this book will address some of these aspects.

BT 3: Integrative Health and Wellbeing Lifestyle: *An Introduction*

In the previous chapter, we discussed some practical considerations and challenges in relation to the Lifestyle interventions from both supply and demand side. In this chapter, we will explore the idea and concept of 'Integrative Health and Wellbeing Lifestyle'.

The ideas and definitions of health, wellbeing, and quality of life have always been a matter of debate and discussion. There are many definitions and indicators from various viewpoints and perspectives. Lack of consensus and consolidation of the vast knowledge that exists in this space raises challenges and prevents their acceptance within the mainstream service delivery.

Exploration of disease-specific life-saving interventions, associated diagnostics, drugs, and vaccines have dominated the picture so far. Lifestyle change, prevention, and health promotion are gaining attention in recent times and have contributed to the evolution of a new branch within modern medicine called Lifestyle Medicine. Great strides are made in the science related to Lifestyle Medicine and many interventions related to diets, physical activity, and stress management are becoming part of clinical practice. How do we best integrate them with other disciplines in order to comprehensively address the 'quality of life' and 'wellbeing dimensions', will need attention.

If we observe the community practices and behaviors, they seem to have found their way. They have never stopped exploring interventions to address their inner wellbeing and quality of life.

Even in developed countries like the U.S. and the U.K., 40-50% of the adult population have accessed one or other non-conventional health-based intervention, either complementary or alternative medicine. They quote the reasons that complementary or alternative medicine offers more autonomy and higher client participation, address lifestyles, and food practices more holistically. Natural products, Yoga, Meditation, and others are some of the common interventions sought.

Complementary medicine refers to adding another discipline with the mainstream, and alternative medicine refers to substituting the conventional with the non-conventional treatment. Often, they are ad-hoc and not scientific. However, integrative health is a new idea that relies on different disciplines working in harmony with each other, informed by evidence and the client's wellbeing. It refers to focusing on the whole person care by bringing together the best of conventional and traditional health approaches in a scientific manner. It focuses on physical, mental, emotional, spiritual, functional, social, and community aspects. Integrative health approaches are explored in the context of pain management, cancers, and specific health behaviors, etc.

While the health industry focuses largely on objective measures of health and wellbeing, and the wellbeing industry (Yoga, Meditation and Ayurveda retreats) focuses on subjective or inner wellbeing. The concept of Integrative Health and Wellbeing brings them both together. A lifestyle that is informed by the modern, as well as traditional disciplines, is referred to as *Integrative Health and Wellbeing Lifestyle.*

The Center for Integrative Health and Wellbeing[1] was set up in order to explore this idea through a review of existing literature as well as through direct practice. The Integrative Health and Wellbeing Lifestyle has its basis in the science and practice of Modern Medicine, Ayurveda, Yoga, and Meditation. A multidisciplinary team of a Physician and a Public Health Specialist, Ayurveda doctors, Yoga Instructor, Meditation trainers, and Lifestyle educators come together in assessing a client of their lifestyle needs, training, and supporting the clients and families in adopting an integrative health and wellbeing lifestyle. All services related to Ayurveda, Yoga, and Meditation are focused on lifestyle modification in complementarity to conventional medicine. The clients are encouraged to keep their primary physician informed of any lifestyle intervention that they receive at the center.

In the next chapter, we will dive deep into the theory, science, and practice of the four disciplines that inform integrative health and wellbeing lifestyle.

---

[1] www.cihw.in

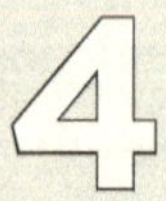

BT 4: Integrative Health and Wellbeing Lifestyle: *Theory and Science*

In the previous chapter, we were introduced to the idea of Integrative Health and Wellbeing Lifestyle. In the current chapter, we will explore the theory, science, and practice of different disciplines that form the basis of Integrative Health and Wellbeing Lifestyle.

BT4A: Modern Medicine (*Lifestyle Medicine*)

The science of Lifestyle Medicine has evolved around a few risk factors (unhealthy behaviors) that are the primary cause of deaths across the world: tobacco consumption, poor diet, physical inactivity, and alcohol consumption. The mechanisms of how these risk factors affect the body physiology giving rise to disease are discussed in the subsequent chapters.

Both in developed and developing countries, it has been hard to change these behaviors. Only 11% of the diabetics in the U.S. followed dietary recommendations in a survey; 40% of a surveyed set of the population in India reported inadequate physical activity. The causes of these behaviors are rooted in industrialization, modern lifestyle, and economic growth.

Studies in Lifestyle Medicine have pointed out the reasons for persisting gaps and also have proposed solutions to address them.

- The physicians are not prioritizing the lifestyle messages or not emphasizing as much as needed. Mere recommendation or prescription of a behavior change has not been helpful.
- Rather, a structured and systematic approach to lifestyle change, engaging the client, and developing an action plan, sound counseling, and follow up support is what makes a difference.
- The role of family and a multidisciplinary team is observed to be critical.
- The physician's competencies in relation to technical knowledge, leadership, and management are highlighted as important for effective practice.

Research shows that the number of healthy behaviors has a direct and inverse relationship with the risk of death, i.e. higher the number, the lower is the risk of dying as a result of any cause.

Individuals who adopted four or more healthy behaviors showed a 66% reduction in mortality rate. These healthy behaviors included regular exercise, not smoking, moderate alcohol consumption, eating healthy, and maintaining optimal body weight. Focusing on healthy lifestyles can avert deaths as well as save costs significantly.

The clustering of these risk factors is observed in adolescence and younger age group, which then continues through adulthood. Thus, targeting preventive efforts in the early years, and at the family level, becomes very critical.

Lifestyle medicine involves the application of environmental, behavioral, clinical, and motivational principles to the management of lifestyle-related health problems. In contrast to conventional medicine, approaches in lifestyle medicine differ considerably, as follows:

- lifestyle causes are the main focus and not treating the risk factors;

- involves long term treatment;
- the patient is an active partner;
- medication is an adjunct to a lifestyle change rather than being the end in itself;
- much emphasis is on motivation and compliance;
- the doctor is a part of the team and not an independent player.

Lifestyle medicine focuses on defining the roots of origin of chronic diseases. It explores causes that are very recent (proximal) as well as remote (distal). For example, risk factor such as high blood pressure has a proximal cause as smoking, a medial cause as stress, and the distal cause as industrialization and modern lifestyle. The following picture that is adapted from Egger et al (2008) illustrates the same.

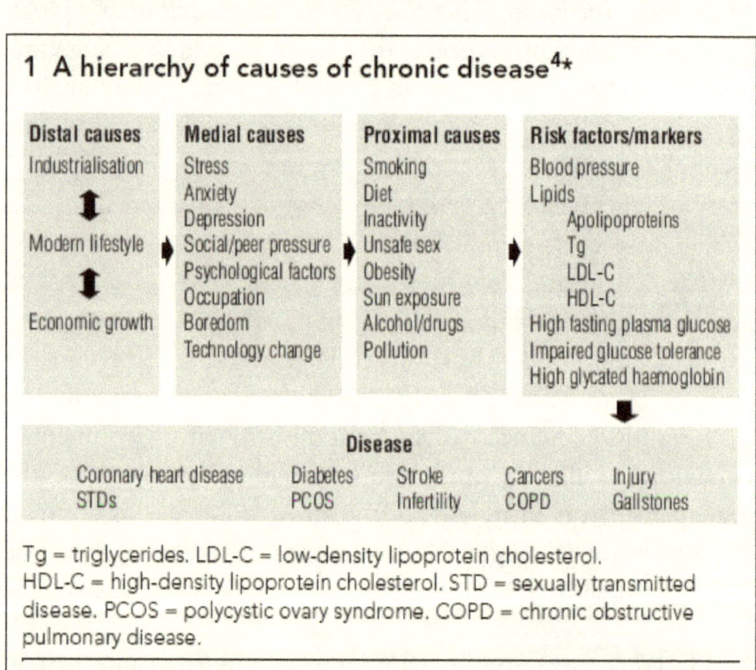

Studies have demonstrated long term benefits of lifestyle medicine in preventing the progress of disease and hence is gaining importance in the current context.

BT4B: Ayurveda

The word Ayurveda comes from the Sanskrit word "Ayu" which means "Life"; and "Veda" which means "Science". It means "Science of Life" and comprises a vast body of knowledge about 'Healthy Living' and 'Treating Disease'. It originated more than 5000 years ago and Charakha, Shusruta, and Vaghbhata are regarded as the first few scholars who described the Ayurveda approaches to healing and wellbeing in detail.

Ayurveda believes that everything in the universe and nature, including every individual, is made of five basic elements- Air, Space, Fire, Water, and Earth.

These elements combine to form three different energies (*Humors* or *Doshas*) that govern the individual's physiological, mental, and emotional build-up and functioning.

- Air and Space combine to form Vata dosha.
- Fire and Water combine to form Pitta dosha.
- Water and Earth combine to form Kapha dosha.

The natural proportion with which these three doshas combine to concoct an individual form the individual's innate constitution (or Prakriti).

Optimal health is achieved when all the three doshas are in equilibrium in accordance with the person's Prakriti. When there is an imbalance in this equilibrium, the condition resulting is known as Vikruti. This results in the setting up of the disease process in an individual's system.

The changes in the constitution are triggered by the following:

- natural factors such as age, time, and seasons
- acquired factors such as changes in foods, lifestyles, thoughts, and emotions.

These changes result in the disturbance of health due to two processes:

- Excess in a particular dosha: This affects the digestive fire leading to improper digestion and metabolism, and leads to the accumulation of undigested metabolic waste, which is referred to as 'Ama'.
- Inadequate and untimely excretion of waste either urine, stool, or sweat (called Mala) also leads to the accumulation of waste in the body, leading to disease.

Hence Ayurveda gives importance to ascertain each individual's original constitution (Prakriti) and its extent of deviation (Vikriti). By techniques of cleansing (detox), lifestyle management, and treatment with medicines, it aims to minimize the deviation to restore health and wellbeing.

The focus of lifestyle education as per Ayurveda is to achieve equilibrium in the constitution. Hence, a dynamic lifestyle is advocated to continuously adapt the body and mind to external changes such as the seasons, life circumstances, and living conditions.

In the recent past, Ayurveda has been researched for its effects on prevention, health promotion, and treatment of diseases. Specific aspects of the lifestyle as per the Ayurveda science and principles will be elucidated in the next section.

BT4C: Yoga

Yoga is a Sanskrit word and has its roots in the "Yuj" which means to connect or balance. It is defined in many ways:

- as a practice that aligns the body, mind, and inner self;
- a way to optimize an individual's fullest potential;
- a tool to expand the individual consciousness into the Universal Consciousness.

Yoga is practiced for different purposes, to improve physical health, to enhance mental wellbeing, and also for achieving spiritual objectives.

Traditionally, Yoga is classified into three types: Jnana Yoga (Path of Knowledge), Karma Yoga (Path of Action), and Bhakti Yoga (Path of Devotion), each supporting and complementing the other. Together, they are believed to assist the practitioner in achieving the higher purpose of human life that transcends physical and mental realms.

Sage Patanjali was one of the first to codify the entire knowledge of Yoga into a system comprising of eight steps, known as Ashtanga (eight-fold) Yoga:

Yama:	removing unwanted habits
Niyama:	acquiring noble qualities
Asana:	refining physical body
Prana:	regulating the breath and life energy
Pratyahara:	drawing the attention inward
Dharana:	Concentration
Dhyana:	Meditation
Samadhi:	Deep absorption

Specific steps and practices were prescribed to a seeker at different stages of the journey towards self-realization.

However today, Yoga is restricted to strengthening the physical body without necessarily harnessing other benefits that it can offer. Often the Yoga postures (asanas) are taught and practiced in a generic way without giving due importance to the subtleties and specifics of practice.

Different postures have different effects on the body and the mind. For example, some postures can reduce blood pressure while some may aggravate it. Hence, the practice of Yoga requires guidance from a skilled trainer and a keen sense of self-observation on part of the practitioner to see if Yoga is yielding the desired goals.

Yoga done systematically under guidance and supervision, in alignment with one's body-mind constitution can have long-lasting benefits at many levels.

Therapeutic Yoga or Yoga Therapy, targeted toward specific disease conditions is an emerging science today. Considerable research is undertaken to study its effects on various chronic diseases such as diabetes and hypertension; mental disorders like depression, anxiety, and stress.

In recent times, it has found acceptance as a complementary approach to conventional treatments to improve wellbeing and quality of life.

Incorporating Yoga as part of one's lifestyle has significant implications for health and wellbeing. Specific postures and breathing exercises have unique effects and if they are aligned to a particular constitution, effects are far-reaching. The subsequent section will throw more light on the same.

BT4D: Meditation

The Cambridge dictionary defines Meditation as "the act of giving one's attention to only one thing, either as a religions activity or as a way of becoming calm and relaxed," or "serious thought or study". It is the translation of the Sanskrit word Dhyana which derives from the root *'Dhyai'* that means *'to contemplate'*.

In the recent past, there has been a growing interest in exploring Meditation for one or other purposes.

What was once sought as a serious practice for spiritual objectives by a select few, is now explored by many, to enhance their health and wellbeing, inner resilience, and productivity.

Research is continuing to shed light on the positive effects of Meditation on health and wellbeing. Increasingly, physicians are recommending Meditation as a complementary tool in the context of mental health issues, and non-communicable diseases such as hypertension.

Studies have shown that Meditation positively affects health and wellbeing across physical, mental, emotional, and spiritual dimensions.

Reduction of blood pressure, regulation of heart rate variability, and the autonomic nervous system, improvement in cardiovascular health are observed. Regulation of stress response, attainment of mental calm, and clarity are experienced by patients with stress, anxiety, and depression. Meditation has also been shown to improve the quality of sleep in patients having sleep disorders.

Positive behaviors and health practices require motivation, self-restraint, and inner resilience that are influenced positively by Meditation. In the context of terminally ill conditions such as advanced cancers, Meditation has shown to result in an inner calm, peace, and acceptance both among the clients and their families.

Thus Meditation not only affects health and wellbeing directly but also influences behaviors and lifestyle changes that improve the quality of life.

Meditation as part of daily routine or lifestyle offers significant benefits in the long run at many levels of wellbeing.

BT4E: Summary - Integrated Model

So far in this chapter we first explored lifestyle medicine from the modern science perspective; later we touched upon how Ayurveda, Yoga, and Meditation influence lifestyle. Thus the integrative health and wellbeing lifestyle that is the focus of this book has a four-prong approach, informed by the four disciplines:

Integrative Health and Wellbeing Lifestyle: four-prong approach

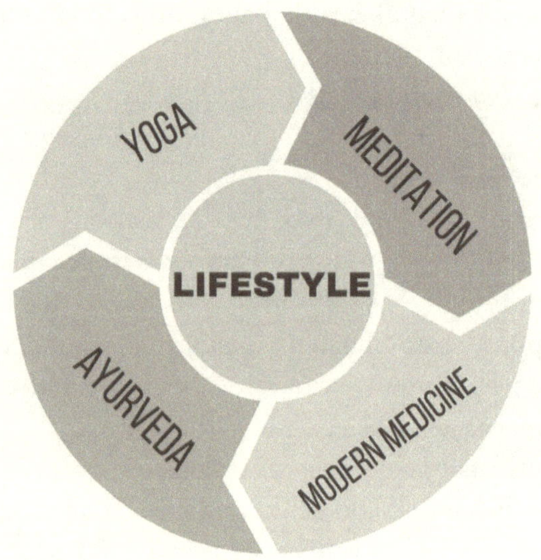

So far in the Background Theory series of this book, we have discussed how the changes in the lifestyle have impacted the health, wellbeing, and quality of life in the current context. We then discussed some challenges and practical considerations in the implementation of lifestyle interventions. Later we explored the idea of integrative health and wellbeing

lifestyle and the four prongs that form its basis: Modern Medicine as Lifestyle Medicine, Ayurveda, Yoga, and Meditation.

In the next section, we will explore each and every component of lifestyle from both a theoretical and practical perspective.

SECTION 2

Preparing for Lifestyle Change: Good to Know (GtK) Series

Here we will cover a series of chapters on various aspects of lifestyle that are important to know. They cover normal physiology and body functioning, patho-physiology in certain disorders due to lifestyle changes, standard lifestyle recommendations as per Modern Medicine, Ayurveda, Yoga, and Meditation.

2.1 Good to Know (GtK): *Lifestyle Medicine Series*

5   GtK 1: Nutrition: *Energy, Metabolism, and Healthy Diet*

*N*utrition *plays a major role in our health and wellbeing as many critical elements that our body requires to be able to function well, come from outside.*

Broadly, nutrition provides two types of nutrients: 1) Macronutrients, that form the bulk of our diets such as carbohydrates, proteins, and fats, and 2) micronutrients, that are required in small fractions such as vitamins and minerals. When they are present in our diet in the right proportion as per our body requirements, we call it a balanced diet. If these nutrients can come from a diverse range of foods – plant and animal sources, fruits and vegetables, it is better.

In the current times, dietary practices have changed due to the change in our lifestyles and living conditions as a result of many factors we discussed earlier.

These faulty dietary practices contribute to many metabolic disorders such as obesity, diabetes, cardiovascular disease, and cancers that we see today. Some of them include:

- Consumption of processed foods;
- Foods high in fats, energy, free sugars, and salt;
- Not eating an adequate amount of vegetables, fruits, or whole grains.

In contrast to balanced diets, these unhealthy food practices fail to meet our energy requirements required for normal metabolism and homeostasis in our body. When this sustains over a prolonged period of time, it begins to affect our health and wellbeing. Hence it is important to fix nutrition as part of our daily routine and lifestyle.

Let us first explore the energy requirements that we have to meet on a day to day basis with the right dietary practices.

In simpler terms, our body organ systems such as cardiovascular (heart and blood vessels) or respiratory (lungs) or nervous system (brain, spinal cord, and nerves), and others require energy continually to function at a certain optimal or basal level. This is called *Basal Metabolic Rate* (BMR) or *Resting Energy Requirement*. Different parts have different energy requirements and the brain has the highest of all.

The overall BMR varies between 1400 and 1800 calories per day and varies by gender.

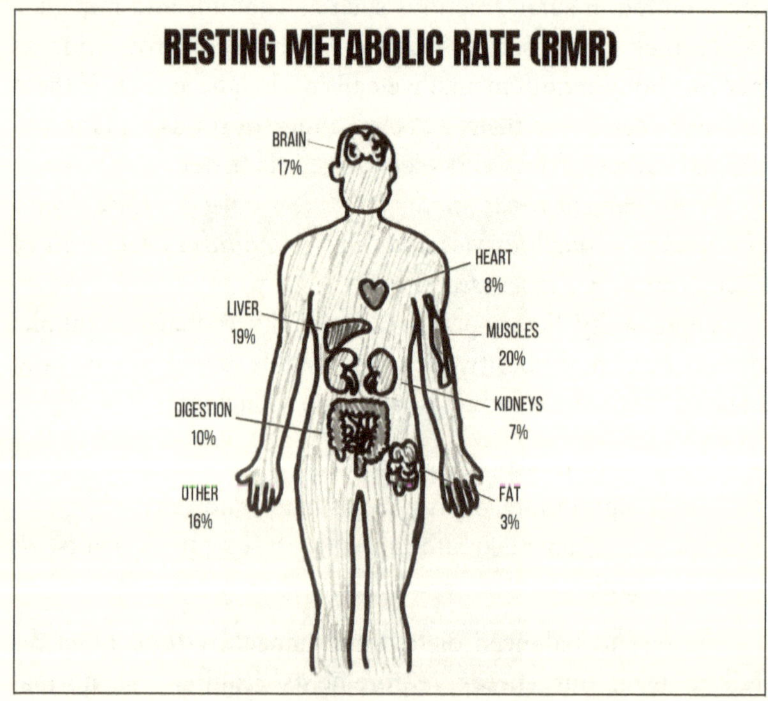

In addition to the resting energy requirement, there are energy requirements to meet the day to day activities.

These energy requirements are largely catered by nutrition. All foods that we consume are broken down into small elements mostly in the stomach and the small intestines: Carbohydrates are broken down into glucose; Proteins into amino-acids and Fats into lipids.

From the small intestine, they are absorbed into the blood and through the circulatory system, they reach all the cells of the body.

In the cells, they go through a series of chemical reactions that release energy.

Excess glucose, amino acids, and lipids will be stored in the body as glycogen, amino-acid pool, and fat stores. During starvation, glucose is regenerated from the breakdown of glycogen (Glycogenolysis) and from amino acids (gluconeogenesis).

Now, let us see how much energy we require for our day to day optimal functioning.

An average adult requires energy to the tune of 2000-2500 kilocalories every day. This helps to maintain the basal metabolic rate at rest as well as to meet additional energy requirements for carrying out external activities.

Those that are involved in strenuous physical activity, need up to 3000 or more kcals/day. These energy requirements vary by gender, age, and physical activity.

The energy requirements are delicately balanced. When energy requirements are sufficiently met, any excess food is stored as glycogen, body proteins, and fats. They are used up during starvation when the body is not receiving food from outside.

Excess intake of energy can result in overweight and obesity that are predisposing risk factors for non-communicable diseases such as diabetes, high blood pressure, stroke, and heart attacks.

A reduced energy intake results in undernutrition and if this persists for long periods, it affects development and functioning.

Now, let us see how a balanced diet helps to meet the required energy.

An ideal balanced diet should be able to meet the energy requirements for:

- activities that continue in the cells and organs during rest (BMR)
- activities over and above BMR, such as physical activity, work, etc.

The macronutrients in the balanced diet are required to meet a certain proportion of the overall energy requirements for optimal body functioning. Carbohydrates, proteins, and fats should contribute to 50-60%, 10-15%, and 30-35% of the energy requirements of our body on a daily basis.

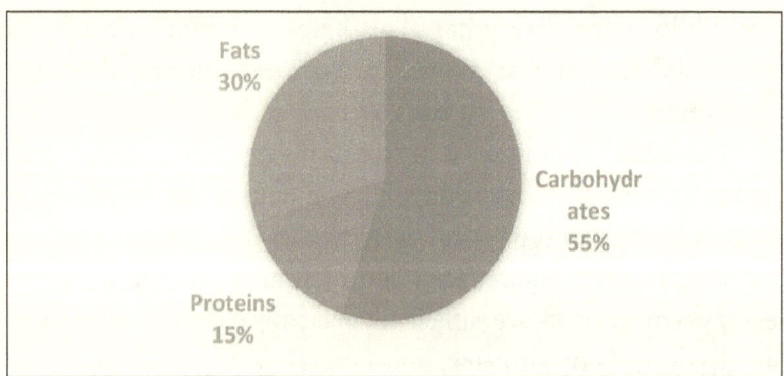

Each of the macronutrients makes a specific energy contribution and this is referred to as *Calorific value*. For carbohydrates, it is 4 kcal (Calories)/gm i.e., one gram of carbohydrate can yield 4 kcals of energy. Similarly, for proteins and fats, these values are 9 and 5, respectively.

For example, a 65 kg man who is moderately active needs about 2500 kcals/day. He should eat about 65 g of protein daily, 95 g of fat, and about 300 g of carbohydrates. Table 1 gives the basis of these calculations:

Nutrition type	% contribution to overall energy intake during the day (a)	Net energy requirement per day (b=a%*2500)	Quantity in grams that will provide energy (b/c)
Carbohydrate	50	1250	300
Protein	15	375	70
Fat	35	875	90

Reference for calculation: 2500 kcal/day energy requirement
A=%energy contribution; b=energy requirement per day due to the food type; c=calorific value (4.1, 9.3, 5.3, respectively for carbohydrates, fats, proteins)

In addition to the energy requirements, certain key cell functions require various minerals and vitamins that should be part of the balanced diet.

Since these are required in very small quantities (micrograms) they are called micronutrients. Despite their requirement in small quantities, their deficiency over long periods will result in certain illnesses. Tables 2 and 3 will refer to the disorders due to their deficiencies. Excess of these minerals also results in toxic symptoms.

#	Mineral	Deficiency
1	Iron	Anemia
2	Cobalt	Anemia
3	Iodine	Thyroid disorders
4	Zinc	Skin ulcers, reduced immunity
5	Copper	Anemia
6	Chromium	Insulin resistance (Diabetes)
7	Fluorine	Dental caries

Vitamins are of two types: fat-soluble that require fats for their absorption (Vitamins A, D, E, K), and water-soluble (B complex, C). Table 3 illustrates the details of the vitamins, their sources, and their deficiency symptoms.

Having explored the basics of nutrition, energy requirements, and balanced diets, macro and micronutrients, let us now review the standard recommendations for a healthy diet.

Healthy Diet Recommendations

- Make whole grains, legumes, and nuts a part of your daily dietary intake. The whole grains should include unprocessed maize, millet, oats, wheat, and brown rice.
- Include at least 400 g or 5 portions of fruit and vegetables as part of your daily diet.
- See that no more than 10% energy intake comes from free sugars (50 g or 12 teaspoons) in a day. Free sugars include all sugars added to foods or drinks, as well as sugars naturally present in honey, syrups, fruit juices and fruit juice concentrates.
- Not more than 30% of total energy should come from fats, preferably should come from unsaturated fats (fish, avocado, nuts, sunflower oil, safflower, soybean, canola, olive oils).

VITAMIN	SOURCES	FUNCTIONS & DEFICIENCIES
A (Retinol)	Milk, Eggs, Carrot, Spinach	Cell differentiation, Vision, Anti-cancer property, immunity, reproductive system development. Deficiency can affect vision, skin, immunity.
B1 (Thiamine)	Wheat, Peas, Beans, Fish, Meats	Breakdown of carbohydrates, proteins and fats; muscle and nerve cell functioning; Deficiency can cause weakness, fatigue, nerve damage, psychosis.
B2 (Riboflavin)	Cheese, Green leafy vegetables, liver, Soybean, almonds.	Converts food to energy, antioxidant; Deficiency can cause fatigue, cracks and sores I the corners of mouth.
B3 (Niacin)	Animal products, nuts, green vegetables, fortified cereals,	Carbohydrate metabolism, functioning of nervous system and digestive system; Deficiency can cause dermatitis, diarrhoea, dementia and sometime death (Pellagra)
B6 (Pyridoxine)	Banana, Potato, Cereals, Yeast, Liver, Fish	Functioning of nervous system and immunity, formation of neurotransmitters, Amino acid synthesis, Red blood cell functioning. Deficiency can cause depression, confusion, irritability, mouth ulcers.
B12	Meat, Fish, Eggs, Yoghurt, Fortified cereals (not adequate from vegetable sources)	Formation of nerve cells and red blood cells. Deficiency can affect nerves and moods.
C	Citrus fruits like orange, grape, lemon; Red peppers, Guava, Broccoli	Growth and repair of tissues, structural part of blood vessels, ligaments and tendons; antioxidant and anticancer properties. Deficiency can cause Scurvy that features as fatigue, mood changes, bleeding gums, decreased immunity.
D	Body produces internally when exposed to sunshine (uv rays for 10 minutes). Other sources are Seafood, Mushrooms, Egg Yolk	Maintain blood levels of calcium and phosphorous; Immunity and growth of bones and teeth. Deficiency in children lead to Rickets (soft and weak bones)
E	Vegetable oils, Nuts, Seeds, Green leafy vegetables.	Cell integrity, antioxidant. Deficiency is rare, and can affect immunity, neuropathy.
K	Spinach, Kale, Turnip, Mustard greens; Soybean, Canola, Olive, Cotton seed oil	Bone growth, Blood coagulation; Deficiency affects clotting and increased bleeding.

- Minimize overall energy intake to less than 10% from saturated fatty acids (fatty meat, butter, palm and coconut oil, cream, cheese, ghee, and lard)
- Avoid trans-fat of all kinds, industrially produced (baked and fried foods, pre-packaged snacks, and foods such as frozen pizza, pies, cookies, biscuits, wafers, and cooking oils and spreads) as well as ruminant trans-fats (meat and dairy foods from ruminant animals such as cows, sheep, goat, and camels)
- Limit the salt intake to less than 5 g per day, from all sources, direct and indirect (snacks and sauces, etc.)
- Increase the intake of potassium that mitigates the negative effects of excess salt (sodium). Potassium is rich in fresh fruits and vegetables.

Practical Action

- *Observe a typical diet that is a part of your current lifestyle. Calculate the energy that it is providing you. Also, list the macronutrients and micronutrients and their contribution to your needs.*
- *From the list of recommendations at the end, pick one healthy recommendation that you can immediately incorporate and one unhealthy practice that you want to eliminate starting this week.*
- *Enter them in your journal, and start working on them, to begin with.*

6 GtK 2: Sleep: *Circadian Rhythm, Biological Clock, and Healthy Sleep*

'*Circa*' means around and 'dies' means day. Cyclical adaptation of our body physiology to the changing rhythm of a 24-hour day-night cycle is Circadian Rhythm.*

They regulate critical functions such as behavior, hormone levels, sleep, body temperature, and metabolism. A mismatch between the external environment and the body rhythm temporarily (as in a jet lag) or over a long time (unhealthy lifestyle) affects health and wellbeing.

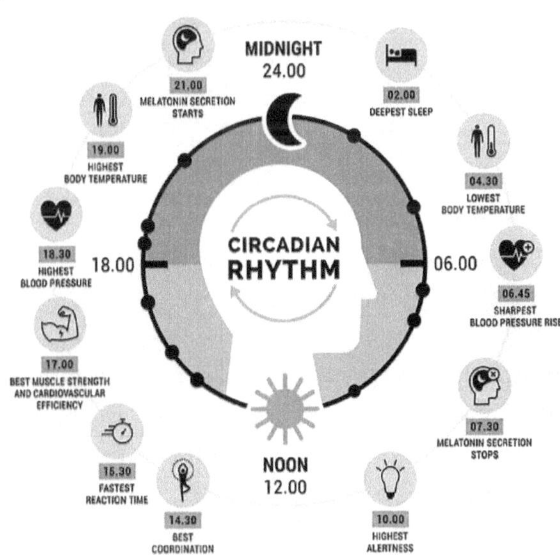

Scientists have isolated specific genes and proteins that oscillate over a 24-hour cycle in response to day-night changes, that influence the circadian rhythm.

These rhythms are discovered in every organ system and are governed by a master circadian pacemaker or a biological clock in the brain. It is particularly located in the hypothalamus and is called Supra-Chiasmatic Nucleus (SCN). SCN is made up of a bundle of 20000 neurons, receives direct input from eyes, and hence is influenced by the light from outside.

Let us see how the Circadian Rhythm is related to Health & Wellbeing.

Circadian Rhythms regulate our sleep cycles through the release of a chemical called melatonin. Melatonin is the hormone that makes one sleepy. It is secreted when there is a reduction in the light coming from the eyes.

So change in day-night cycles, shift working conditions, or exposure to excess light from gadgets can affect sleep cycles.

Circadian Rhythms also affect hormone release, eating habits, digestion, body temperature, and other bodily functions. Changes in these rhythms give rise to chronic health conditions such as sleep disorders, obesity, diabetes, and mental health issues.

Circadian Rhythm disturbances also affect the secretion of certain cytokines that are critical for immune response and thus affect the body's immunity.

Circadian Rhythm has a strong relationship with food intake.

Research shows that Circadian Rhythms are affected by both the quality and quantity of the food we take, as well as the daily eating pattern.

Studies have shown that despite consuming an identical quantity of the meal for breakfast and dinner, there was a higher rise in blood glucose after dinner; it also persisted for a longer duration than after breakfast. This is because of melatonin which suppresses insulin secretion from the pancreas. Insulin is responsible to clear the glucose from the blood soon after the meals.

Hence adapting dietary habits to these Circadian Rhythms have implications for controlling metabolic disorders.

Research shows that if feeding is restricted to within 10 hours; for example: break the fast at 7:00 am in the morning and take the other two meals or snacks within the next 10 hours. This is also known as **time-restricted feeding**; it has shown to result in a reduction of weight and can improve sleep.

Overnight fasting over 13 hours has shown to improve the prognosis of breast cancer as well as prevent breast cancer.

Studies also indicate that early eaters are more prone to weight loss than late eaters.

Sleep and Wellbeing

Sleep time is a time of rest and repose to the body and mind. Sufficient quantity and quality of sleep will recharge the body to take up the activities during the day. In the recent past, there is a greater understanding of what happens in sleep and how sleep contributes to health and wellbeing in a significant way.

Lifestyles affect sleep and indirectly the health and wellbeing

Sleep research shows that the current lifestyles characterized by altered work styles, food practices, and stress have disrupted sleep cycles. Chronic sleep disturbance can result in medical disorders such as diabetes, obesity, stroke, sleep disorders, and mental health issues.

Let us understand these sleep cycles a little bit more.

Every adult requires a fixed number of hours of sleep in the range of 6-8 hours. During sleep, one goes through two phases: a phase where there are no eye movements (non-rapid eye movement; NREM sleep) and a phase of rapid eye movements (REM sleep).

NREM sleep has further stages based on brain activity that is detected through electroencephalogram (EEG). EEG is a graphic representation of brain activity similar to an electrocardiogram for the heart.

- In stage 1 of NREM, a person is transitioning from wakefulness to a sleepy state. High-frequency waves are the characteristic feature of the EEG.
- In stage 2, the sleep sets in. In an EEG, sleep onset is detected as spindles and K complexes against backdrop low-frequency waves.
- In stage 3, the person is in the deepest stage of sleep; brain activity is lowest, and the muscles are completely relaxed and immobile. This is also called slow-wave sleep (SWS) as the EEG picks up high amplitude and low-frequency slow waves (< 5 Hz, referred to as delta frequency)

Earlier NREM stages 3 and 4 were identified as two different phases, but now they are clubbed together. NREM stage 3 is followed by the REM phase of sleep, and then the NREM stages 1 to 3 will repeat in a cyclical manner.

When a person is woken up during the REM stage of sleep, he can recall the dreams.

In an average sleep duration of 6-7 hours, an adult goes through the cycle of NREM stages 1-2-3-REM about 4-6 times, each cycle lasting 80 to 110 minutes. Stage 3 is particularly important in the context of health and wellbeing, where a person spends about 20 min in each cycle.

In stage 3, the whole body is rejuvenated at the cellular level; the immune process is regenerated and cellular level detoxification is detected.

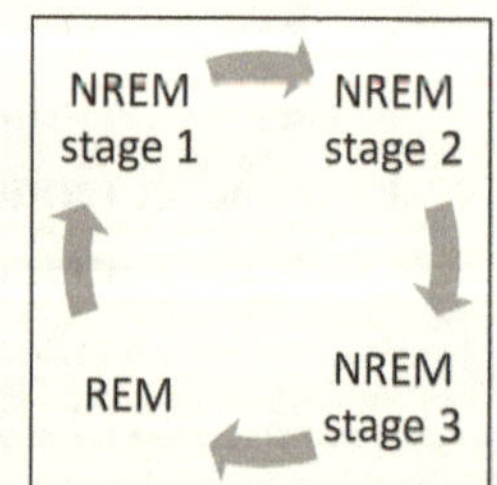

However, when sleep cycles are disrupted due to altered lifestyles, a person does not get his or her required duration of deep sleep. Stage 3 is reduced both in frequency and duration.

Sleep studies have shown that sleep disturbance results in the release of stress hormones that induce secretion of pro-inflammatory cytokines and tumor necrosis factors. These changes when sustained for long periods are implicated in inflammatory disorders such as cardiovascular disease, cancer, depression, infectious disease, etc.

Various lifestyle aspects such as working conditions, travel, food practices, substance use, etc. are implicated in sleep disruption in adults.

Even among the children, the widespread use of electronic gadgets is affecting sleep cycles in many ways: excess light exposure, psychological stimulation, heightened alertness, etc. Childhood obesity, impaired cognitive and academic functioning, and disturbed psychological wellbeing are reported by studies.

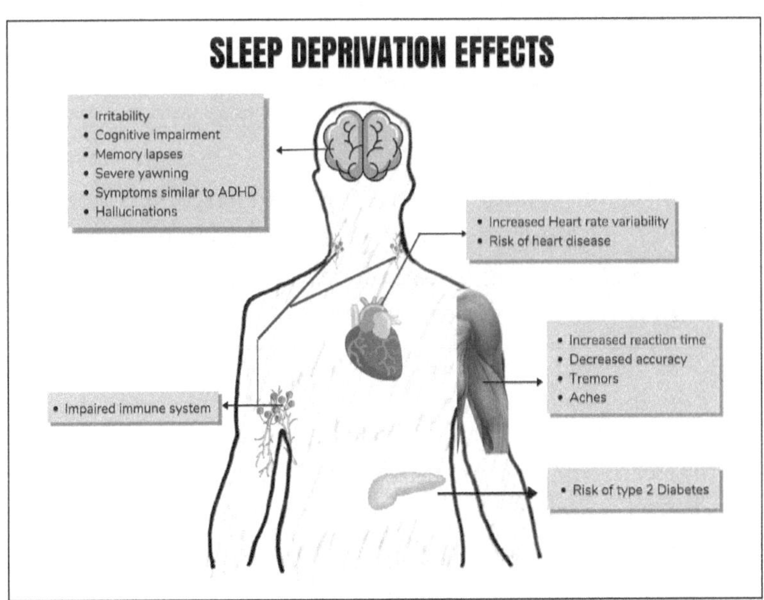

Lifestyle recommendations to improve sleep and wellbeing:

- A number of lifestyle changes have shown to impact the quality of sleep and indirectly health and wellbeing as well.
- Fix your time to go to bed at night and to wake up in the morning. This helps to establish rhythm and discipline.
- Align your sleep cycle with natural cycles of day and night. Studies have shown that shift workers who cannot adhere to a certain rhythm are more prone to metabolic disorders.
- Minimize the light exposure to the eyes in the late evenings and particularly an hour or two before going to bed. Particularly pay attention to the radiation and light emission from the gadgets, television, computers, etc. and minimize it.
- Dim light of particular frequencies can calm the mood and help to sleep well.
- Eat lightly for dinner. Keep a gap of two hours between dinner and sleep. The meal during dinner time results in higher blood glucose levels than at other times. This influences glucose metabolism and secretion of melatonin hormone that is responsible for sleep.
- Relaxation and Meditation in the evenings help to calm the mind. Brains show more relaxed states (low-frequency waves on EEG) during meditation that is conducive to good sleep.
- Avoid any emotional or intellectual exchange in the late hours before going to bed, as they heighten brain activity and slow down the sleep cycles.
- Avoid stimulants such as caffeine and nicotine, late in the evening.
- Soft and relaxing music can calm the mind and prepare it for sleep. Music entrainment is a well-studied phenomenon where the music of a particular frequency can entrain the brains into resonating at the same frequency. Alpha (low wave) entrainment has informed many brain training

programs that aim at calming and relaxing the children to optimize their performance.

- Reading a book of one's interest is a good practice at the end of the day. It keeps one away from the gadgets and helps to switch to sleep.
- Physical activity, Yoga, and work-outs can stretch the body muscles, facilitate circulation, and aid in good sleep.
- If sleep problems persist and affect your performance, it is a good idea to see a physician and have an assessment done.

Practical Action

- *Observe the pattern of your sleep. Note down the following in your diary: sleep duration, number of times you woke up, how you feel when you wake up in the morning.*
- *Start with a few changes from the above recommendations: take two at a time and gradually adopt the others. Continue to document their effects on your sleep quantity and quality.*
- *Every time you make/add a lifestyle change, try to correlate its effects on your sleep.*

7 GtK 3: Physical Activity: *Physiology, Benefits, and Recommendations*

In the current days, a sedentary lifestyle is a common feature due to changing work culture and living conditions.

Studies show that inadequate physical activity increases the chances of overweight, obesity, diabetes, cardiovascular disease, cancer, etc. by 15-20% and reduces lifespan by 3-5 years.

WHO indicates that inadequate physical activity is a modifiable risk factor that should be addressed sufficiently as part of lifestyle education in all age groups. Several research studies have documented that adopting physical activity as part of a lifestyle can prevent many diseases while promoting health and wellbeing.

Let us understand the terms: Physical Activity and Exercise

Any bodily activity that involves skeletal muscle contraction and expenditure of energy is called physical activity. It may include a range of activities: walking, cycling, swimming, running, exercises, sports, work out in a gymnasium, Yoga, etc.

Exercise is one of the physical activities that involves planned, structured, repetitive movements, aimed to improve physical fitness.

Exercise has the following effects on the body:

- Heart and blood vessels: Increases cardiac output, blood pressure, and blood flow to the muscles

- Lungs: increases ventilation in the lungs and exchange of gases
- Skeletal muscles: helps in growth, repair, and regeneration of skeletal muscles through increasing mitochondrial activity, gas exchange in the cells
- Mood: stimulates the release of chemicals (endorphins) that elevate mood and positivity
- Hormones: stimulates the release of growth hormone that enhances bone and tissue growth
- Blood glucose: long term exercise increases insulin sensitivity and helps to regulate blood glucose
- Blood cholesterol: increases good cholesterol (also known as HDL – high-density lipoprotein cholesterol) and reduces bad cholesterol (LDL – low-density lipoprotein)
- Cell nourishment: supplies nutrition and oxygen to cells
- Immunity: boosts immunity, reduces inflammation
- Brain: induces brain neuroplasticity (neuronal connections)

Hence, the following benefits are accorded:

- Strengthens the muscles
- Improves cardiac fitness
- Improves lung capacity
- Improves functional health (movement of body parts due to bones, joints, muscles, nerves, etc.; also called mechanical wellbeing)
- Reduces the risk of many diseases: obesity, diabetes, stroke, cancers, etc.
- Helps to expend energy and maintain energy balance
- Improves flexibility of the body
- Improved mood and cognition
- Improves quality of life

Experts recommend four different types of exercises for a holistic body and mind development.

Aerobic exercises: They increase heart rate, breathing, and endurance. 150 minutes of moderate-intensity exercise is recommended. Swimming, brisk walking, jogging, cycling, dancing, etc.

Strength training: This helps to build muscle mass and restores against the loss of muscle that is a process of normal aging. This will build confidence in dealing with day to day activities, especially in the elderly age.

Stretching: Stretching improves the length of muscles, flexibility, and range of motion. With aging, muscles and tendons lose flexibility, muscles shorten and weaken resulting in cramps, pains, muscle damage, strains, joint pain, and falls.

Balance: These exercises help to maintain steadiness in body stance and prevent falls, especially in the aged who are prone to falls due to natural degeneration of nerves involved in balance – vision, inner ear, brain, muscles, and joints, etc.

Physical activity is recommended for all age groups in different formats.

Children and Adolescents (5 to 17 years)

At least 60 minutes or greater of moderate to vigorous-intensity activity daily.

Activities that strengthen muscle and bone, at least three times a week.

Adults (18 to 64 years)

At least 150 minutes of moderate intensity activity or 75 minutes of vigorous-intensity activity throughout the week.

For additional benefits, 300 minutes of moderate intensity activity throughout the week.

Activities to strengthen major muscles, at least twice a week.

Adults aged 65 years and above

The above activities mentioned for adults are applicable here also but should be planned after considering mobility and flexibility.

Those with poor mobility should perform physical activity (three or more times a week) to enhance balance and prevent falls.

Practical Action

- *Observe the pattern of your physical activity and exercises. Are you able to do all four types? If not, what is missing?*
- *Add the missing element. Observe the effect on the body and mind and document them.*
- *If you are a beginner, start with anyone. Start with a small duration and slowly increase the duration over a period of time.*

8   GtK 4: Tobacco and Alcohol: *Effects, Physiology, and Healthy Recommendations*

Tobacco and alcohol consumption has become part of a routine of millions across the world for various reasons: exploration, stress, socializing, social status, habituation, and dependence.

Tobacco causes 8 million deaths; and alcohol causes 3 million deaths globally each year. WHO lists them as unhealthy lifestyle practices and suggests healthy recommendations to maintain health and wellbeing.

Health Risk With Tobacco and Alcohol Use

Tobacco is a major risk factor for cardiovascular and respiratory diseases (chronic obstructive pulmonary disease), and up to 20 different types of cancers (lung, throat, pancreas, kidneys, leukemia, etc.). It can raise blood pressure and cholesterol levels, reduce bone density, increase the risk of infertility, pre-term delivery, still-birth, and sudden death in infants.

Alcohol use has toxic effects on the cardiovascular system, the digestive system, is linked with cancer, suppresses the immune system, and increases the risk of Tuberculosis and HIV. Alcohol has interaction with medications; heavy drinking leads to intoxication, nausea and vomiting, blurred vision, impaired judgment, alcohol poisoning, and accidental injuries.

Long term alcohol use causes high blood pressure, gastric disease, liver cirrhosis, liver cancer, pancreatitis, memory and cognition problems, alcohol dependence, and psychological conditions.

Both lead to premature deaths and disability of productive age among adults.

Studies have shown that one can influence the other; for example, nicotine exposure can promote alcohol dependence thus increasing the risk of a multitude of health problems.

How Tobacco Affects Health

All forms of tobacco use pose risk and cigarette smoking is the most common form of its consumption. Cigarettes contain up to 4000 chemical compounds and toxic agents including carbon monoxide, tar, DDT, arsenic, and formaldehyde which are carcinogenic.

These chemicals and additives disrupt the respiratory protective lining and suppress the local immunity. Smoking also causes inflammation and pre-cancerous changes.

Chronic smoking results in obstruction of respiratory passage (chronic obstructive pulmonary disease - COPD) and reduces lung capacity.

Smoking increases heart rate, blood pressure, and metabolic rate.

Nicotine raises the resting metabolic rate but blunts the expected increase in food intake in response to raised metabolic rate. This leads to reduced body weight. These effects are mediated through its effects on the brain and endocrine system.

Nicotine has a high potential for addiction through its effects on the reward system of the brain. With repeated exposure, tolerance develops and hence brain will need greater amounts of nicotine for achieving satiety.

How Alcohol Affects Health

Similar to Nicotine and other addictive substances, alcohol also influences the brain's reward circuitry system and release of dopamine that is associated with behavioral motivation and reward.

Alcohol (Ethanol) metabolism will result in products that are toxic to cells; they can damage cellular proteins and cause cell death; they can induce changes in metabolism and cellular respiration.

Chronic alcohol will cause damage to the lining of the digestive tract causing inflammation and bleeding.

Reduced oxidation of fatty acids and metabolic changes in the liver will lead to fat accumulation – fatty liver, infection (hepatitis), and cirrhosis.

High consumption for prolonged time periods will lead to a rise in blood pressure, higher heart rate, arrhythmias, and heart failure also.

Alcohol dependence can lead to nerve degeneration (including cerebellum) that affects gait, stance, tingling, and numbing sensation of hands and feet.

Expert Recommendations to Control Tobacco and Alcohol Consumption

Awareness of effects and health hazards is always the best place to start, irrespective of whether someone is already exposed or not.

Public health recognizes different levels of prevention at every stage of manifestation of a lifestyle disease:

- **Primordial prevention:** here, prevention starts very early even before the occurrence of the disease or the risk factor that predisposes to the disease (such as tobacco and alcohol use). Efforts and education start during childhood.

- **Primary prevention:** here, risk factor (alcohol or tobacco use) has already emerged and the focus is to prevent the occurrence of disease (hypertension or diabetes) through appropriate lifestyle change and risk control (reduction of frequency or complete stoppage).
- **Secondary prevention:** here, the disease has already occurred and the focus is the prevention of complications through medication and lifestyle management. In the example of diabetes, the patient should be treated with anti-diabetic medications and appropriate lifestyle change (diets, exercise, reduction of tobacco or alcohol, etc.).
- **Tertiary prevention:** here, complications have already occurred and the focus is limited to rehabilitation and restoring quality of life to the best possible levels.

Secondary and tertiary prevention aren't truly prevention as the disease and complications have already set in. Yet, what is assuring is that all stages can be managed to achieve the most optimal outcome for any stage.

Here are a few recommendations and tips toward controlling alcohol and tobacco use at a personal level:

- For someone engaged in both, best is to focus on one problem at a time and disrupt the connection between the two.
- Reduce a little each day; one less cigarette or drink each day.
- Step up other activities; Yoga, sports, and workout.
- Plan social meetings in non-smoking and non-alcoholic zones.
- Specific to smoking, a gradual reduction method or delay methods (postponing cigarettes as much as possible) have been found effective.

- Abrupt cessation, popularly known as a cold turkey is also effective in many instances.
- Support of family members and friends plays an important role; plan along with them.
- Meditation and calming techniques bring in the pause, restraint, and self-control and help to get over the habits.
- In cases of a high degree of dependence medication and behavior modification, therapy will be required.

There is no one single magic bullet, and one has to choose methods that work best, practically. Strong motivation and determination is the key.

Practical Action

- *Note down your current status: how frequently and how much do you smoke or drink in a day and week, respectively?*
- *From within the recommendations, can you pick one or two for smoking and alcohol? You can start with either of them.*

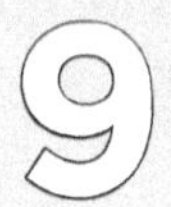

GtK 5: Stress and Immunity: *Effects, Physiology, and Healthy Behaviors*

Stress is a universal phenomenon in current times and no age group or profession or place is spared.

The growing number of suicides and various mental health issues year after year, both in the young and the old, from developed and developing countries, in urban and rural areas are a testimony to this fact. Stress is implicated in many metabolic and mental health issues and it has generated a great deal of interest as part of lifestyle medicine, to explore its neuro-behavioral mechanisms for effective management.

Stress, Eustress, and Distress

Stress is a natural body-mind response to any change in the environment, either internal or external.

The brain, endocrine glands, and various body systems come together in the play to respond to a stimulus. 'Stress response' as it is known, has existed in all times and life-forms and has been responsible for the survival of the old stone age man. Thus stress, in its fundamental nature, is protective and useful. This is also known as good stress or 'Eustress'. Eustress improves focus and performance.

However, when stress exceeds a certain threshold and overrides its protective value and harms the body and mind, it is called bad stress or 'Distress'. This is popularly known as simply stress and has many implications for health and wellbeing.

Stress, Disease, and Lifestyles

Studies have shown that persistent stress over months and years, can affect various body systems. This gives rise to diseases such as obesity, overweight, and sometimes underweight, hypertension, diabetes, stroke, cancer, etc.

Mental health issues such as depression, anxiety, suicides, and breakup in relationships at home and workplaces, poor performance and productivity, are also attributed to stress.

Changing lifestyles, living conditions as a result of globalization, urbanization, work culture, etc. are responsible for the distress and its effects, that we witness today.

Minds are processing a lot more information than before with the explosion of information technology and social media. The careers are displacing individuals and families from their roots, culture, base locations, and native lifestyles. Transitioning from a joint family to the nuclear family systems has reduced coping abilities at homes too. Boundaries between work-life and home-life are getting thinner that is eroding the relationships which otherwise would have been the shock-absorber of stress.

Physiology of Stress: Fight or Flight Response

As said earlier, the stress response is a natural response mediated through the body's neuro-endocrine system with the sole objective of protection and survival.

Every time there is a threat in the form of an external stimulus, the complex network of connections and communication between the pre-frontal cortex (which deals with executive functions), hippocampus (memory), amygdala (fear perception), and hypothalamus (stress response through H-P-A axis) are involved.

Stress response starts with the release of Corticotrophin releasing hormone (CTH) by the hypothalamus. CTH signals the pituitary gland to release a chemical (ACTH, adreno-cortico-trophic hormone) into the blood, which in turn stimulates adrenal glands (situated on the top of the kidneys) to release another hormone (Cortisol) into the blood.

This complex mediation between hypothalamus-pituitary-adrenal glands is known as the H-P-A axis. Cortisol, also known as **stress hormone** stimulates the release of two hormones from the adrenal gland: adrenaline and noradrenaline which are responsible for various responses that are outlined below.

These two hormones are also released as a result of the stimulation of the sympathetic nervous system directly by the hypothalamus upon perceiving fear.

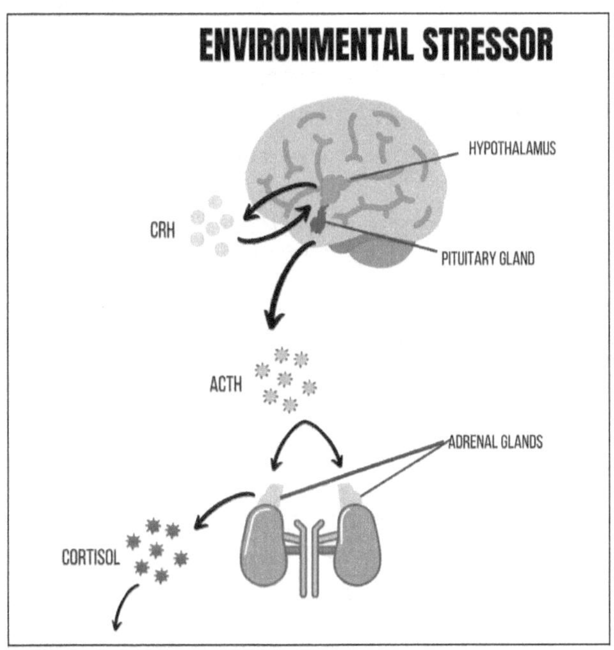

The sympathetic and parasympathetic nervous systems form part of the peripheral autonomic nervous system (outside of the brain and spinal cord, and are responsible for various functions of internal organs like heart, lungs, kidney, etc.).

The sympathetic and parasympathetic nervous systems have opposite effects; the former prepares the body to react during stress and the latter keeps the body in a relaxed state.

The sympathetic nervous system mediates its effects through the two hormones: adrenaline and noradrenaline that have effects on various parts of the body.

- They stimulate contraction of the heart and the large blood vessels, thus increasing blood pressure and diverting blood flow to the skeletal muscles, to enable fleeing away from the scene.
- They stimulate the contraction of the lungs and facilitate a faster exchange of gases required for higher metabolism in the cells needed in stressful situations.
- They control insulin secretion, and stimulate glycogen from the pancreas, eventually rising blood glucose that is required to meet higher energy needs during these instances.

Thus, this stress response is characterized by an increase in heart rate, rise in blood pressure, rapid breathing, rise in blood glucose, increased nourishment to the muscles, all geared up toward helping an individual either to face or run away from the scene of danger. Hence, it is also called 'fight or flight' response.

Stress and the Immune System

The immune system is the natural defense of the body against infections. Immunity is the ability of the body to protect itself from any injury or infection. This is mediated through certain types of cells and mechanisms. Several factors influence the

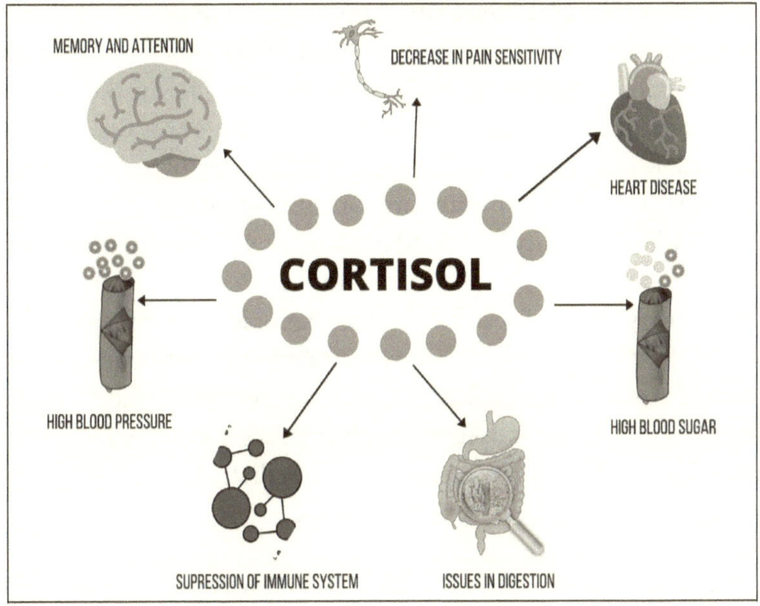

strength of Immunity: genetic makeup, nutrition, exercise, physical and mental wellbeing, exposure to toxins and infections, etc. Environmental factors such as age, gender, and even seasonal changes are also implicated. Here, we will particularly discuss how stress impacts immunity and makes the body vulnerable to diseases.

Let us first explore the physiology of Immunity and the Immune response system.

Immunity can be broadly classified into three types: Innate, Active (Adaptive or Acquired), and Passive Immunity.

Innate Immunity exists right from the time of birth. It forms the first line of defense of the body for skin or mucous surface of the gut.

Active Immunity is triggered in response to an infection. Antibodies are produced by the body to fight against an invading organism. When this happens as a result of a disease, it is called **Natural Immunity**. This can be induced by vaccines when it is called **Vaccine-induced Immunity**. Active Immunity is generally long-lasting and sometimes for life. In the future when the same organism invades again, the body remembers it and produces the antibodies to fight the organism. This phenomenon is called **Immunological Memory**.

Passive Immunity is referred to as instances when the Immunity is transferred from one person to another. The individual's Innate Immune system is not involved. For example, the newborn baby in the first few months is protected due to the antibodies that it carries from the mother. Antibodies can be transferred through blood products as is done through Immune globulins in certain conditions. Here the protection is immediate, but it lasts for a short duration, a few weeks to months.

Blood cells in the blood, also called Leucocytes, are mainly involved in the immune response.

The Leucocytes are produced in the Thymus, Spleen, Bone marrow, and Lymph nodes, which are known as Lymphoid organs. They produce cells that float in the blood and are constantly on the watch. Two types of cells are involved in the immune response:

Phagocytes: they surround the microbes, break them down, and eat them; this process is known as Phagocytosis. They are of many types with different functions, for example, Neutrophils that attack bacteria; Macrophages that remove dead cells and debris; Mast cells that assist in healing wounds.

Lymphocytes: they remember the microbes and recognize them when they again attack the body (Immunological Memory). They are of two types: B lymphocytes that produce antibodies against pathogens; and T lymphocytes that destroy compromised cells in the body.

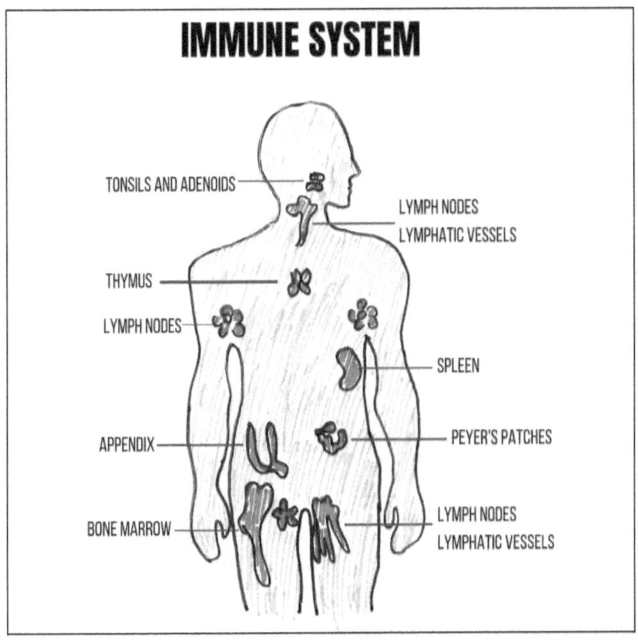

Now let us understand how the immune response takes place.

The immune system is triggered by the entry of an antigen (virus, bacteria, fungus, or the dead cells within the body). B lymphocytes produce antibodies that then attack the antigen. They lock or mark the antigen and make it available for the kill by the phagocytes. Antibodies are of many types and functions:

Immunoglobulin G or IgG – marks the antigens
IgM – attacks bacteria
IgA – is present in fluids like saliva, tears
IgE – against parasites and allergies
IgD – is bound to B lymphocytes and helps to trigger the immune response

T lymphocytes are of 2 types that act in different ways. Helper T cells coordinate immune response and Killer T cells attack the compromised cells.

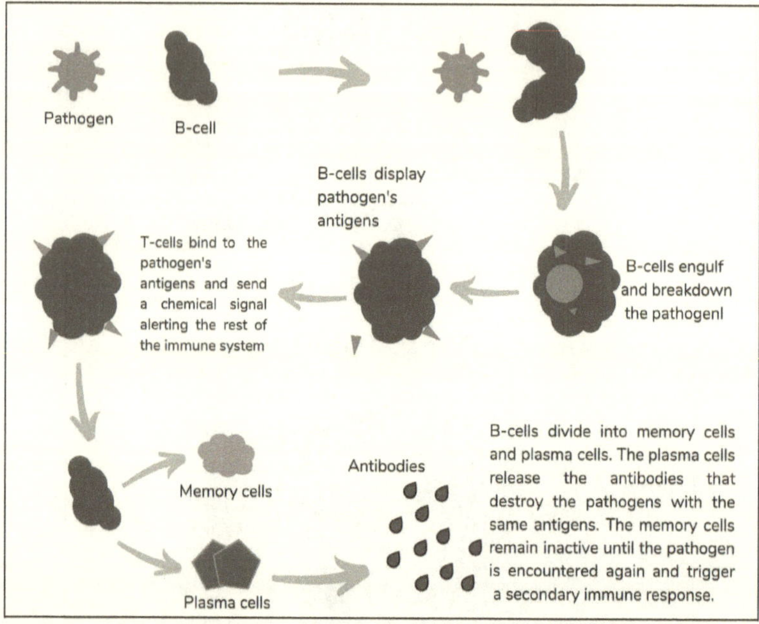

Having understood the basics about immunity and immune response, let us review some recent research findings as to how stress affects immunity.

We previously discussed how stress response stimulates cortisol production and the sympathetic nervous system, which eventually affects several body systems including immunity.

The lymphoid organs such as bone marrow, thymus spleen, lymph nodes are supplied by sympathetic nerve fibers. During a stress response, these fibers release chemicals that bind to the white blood cells (leucocytes) and influence immune response.

Both acute stress and chronic stress influence immune response.

Acute episodes of stress elicit a 'fight or flight' response. The cells are redistributed to prepare the natural immune system for an immune response. It is as if the cells are anticipating any injury or infection. This adaptive ability will decrease when stress becomes chronic.

In long-standing stressful situations such as bereavement or trauma, it is observed that the natural killer cell effects are reduced in their strength. T cells are reduced in number in the blood circulation.

Studies have documented that during the annual examinations, medical students showed reduced natural killer cells, that usually fight tumor cells and viral infections. Childhood stress has shown to result in long-lasting physical and mental health wellbeing issues.

More recent evidence shows that stress induced inflammation can increase the likelihood of developing a disease or exacerbation of an existing disease. This is observed in autoimmune conditions such as rheumatoid arthritis and chronic inflammatory conditions such as irritable bowel syndrome (IBD).

So far we have covered information about stress and how it affects our health and wellbeing. Now, let us explore simple and effective steps to combat stress

Experts suggest the following recommendations that can help deal with stress:

- Be aware of the positive and negative effects of stress.
- Acceptance of the fact that stress is universal and none is spared, and self-belief that it can be managed, goes a long way in building resilience.
- Clarity and focus can help alleviate stress. Meditation, breathing exercises, and relaxation techniques have shown a reduction in stress levels effectively in many studies.
- Music, journal writing, dialogue with a friend (or a mentor).
- Yoga, workout, and sports as part of lifestyle mitigate stress and can also strengthen the mindset.
- When stress is persisting or overwhelming and starts affecting day-to-day activities, it is time to take professional help from a counselor or a physician.

Practical Action

- *Stress can be quantified and several scales are available.*
- *From the list of recommendations start 2-3 activities and explore their impact on your stress levels.*

2.2 Good to Know (GtK):
Ayurveda Series

10 GtK 6: Individual's Unique Body-Mind Constitution: *An Introduction*

*A*yurveda school of thought that all matter in this universe is made up of five basic elements.

These elements, namely Ether, Air, Fire, Water, and Earth, combine to form the three types of energies called Vata, Pitta, and Kapha. These energies are known as the *Humors* or *Doshas*.

The combination of these three energies results in a unique body-mind constitution of every individual. All the physiological and psychological activities are attributed to the functioning of these energies in various combinations and intensity.

Let us explore each of them and their characteristics.

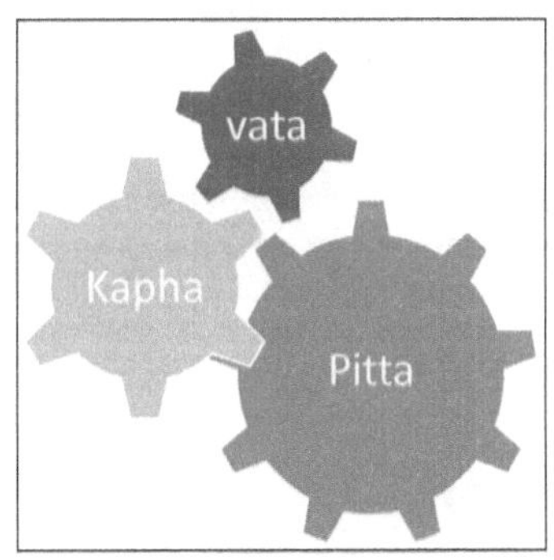

VATA

- The Vata dosha is composed of air and ether. It is characterized by the properties of movement, dryness, and lightness just as those elements.
- It is responsible for all the functional movements in the body and mind such as:
  - at the bodily level - heartbeat, blood flow, neural currents;
  - and at the mind level - thinking process, creativity, agility, etc.

- While the energy expands across the body and mind, it has its seat in the colon (large intestine).
- This is the subtlest and most mobile of all the three energies. Hence aggravation of this energy easily impacts the other two as well and upsets the overall balance in the constitutional build-up.

PITTA

- The Pitta dosha is a combination of the fire and the water elements and is characterized by sharpness, heat, and pungency.
- It is responsible for all the transformative processes:
    o   at bodily level - digestion of food, metabolic activities, etc.;
    o   at mind level - assimilation of knowledge, intelligence, etc.
- Pitta is also mobile in nature. It influences the quality of blood and of vision among other things.
- Its seat is the small intestine whose primary task is the assimilation of food.
- When in balance, Pitta aids in good metabolism. When out of balance, it results in digestive disorders, skin disorders, inflammatory disorders, etc.

KAPHA

- The Kapha dosha is the combination of the earth and the water elements. Much as in these elements, the qualities of steadiness, heaviness, sliminess, and viscosity characterize the Kapha dosha.
- This is responsible for giving structure, stability, lubrication, and protection to the body and forms the muscles and bones. It holds the cells together and is responsible for the healing aspect of the body as well as its immunity.
- Chest is the main seat of Kapha dosha in the body.

- When in balance, it enables the stability and strength of the body and steadiness of mind and good memory. When aggravated and out of balance, it results in congestion, allergies, sluggishness, the heaviness of body and mind, and lethargy among other things.

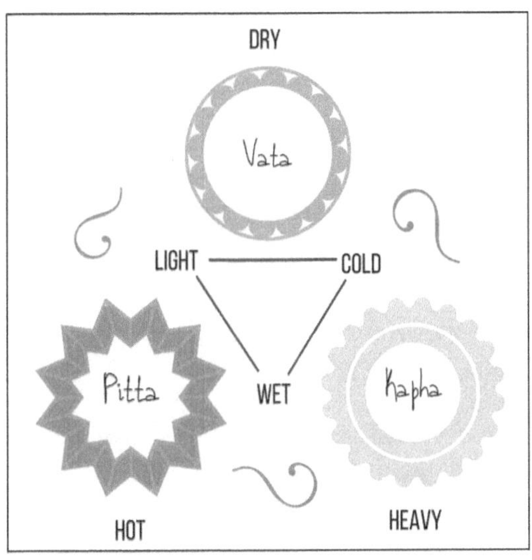

Various factors decide the formation of the Individual Constitution.

The Individual Constitution is decided even before the birth of the baby, and at the time of conception. It is influenced by the constitution of the parents, time of the day, quality of the season, etc. The original or natural body constitution is called *Prakriti.*

After the birth and while growing up, one or two of the doshas in the constitution acquires dominance, resulting in a specific type of constitution for that person. In this way, a person can have a predominantly Vata or Pitta or Kapha type of constitution.

Each of the constitutional types has several defining characteristics at the physical, mental, and emotional levels.

This means that the person's body and mind tend to be behaving in line with the doshic dominance prevalent in his constitution. For example, a Vata type person can tend to be very creative or restless owing to the nature of Vata dosha.

More commonly, the constitutional makeup of a person will have the dominance of two doshas such as the Vata-Pitta type or the Kapha-Pitta type, etc. The first mentioned dosha is more defining in the characteristics of that person.

The details of various characteristics for each of the doshas are provided in the annexure.

How does this knowledge help?

Wellbeing recommendations provided by the Ayurveda are specific to the constitutional makeup of the individual. While standard guidelines do have relevance at a physical and physiological level, Ayurveda adds value considering the unique requirements of the individual based on their constitution.

The recommendations are dynamic as well. Based on the changes in external factors such as seasons or place that may influence the constitution, Ayurveda recommends changes in lifestyles and food practices accordingly.

By responding to the self-assessment questionnaire in the annexure, you will have a fair idea of your basic constitution. This when complemented by the pulse examination (*Naadi pareeksha*) by an Ayurveda physician, completes the assessment.

Practical Action

- *Identify four to five physical features in you and try to relate to a particular dosha.*

- *Study your general inner temperament and try to relate to a corresponding doshic component.*
- *Do not arrive at a conclusion based on just a few parameters, but explore all the parameters and what dominates the pattern. You may even use this on 2-3 different occasions, also ask your close friend or partner to do this and slowly arrive at an inference. Rightly done, you can assess your present constitution (deviated form) as well as what generally dominates (original constitution).*
- *Observe three or four people in your close circle and try to assess their constitution type based on their physical, mental, and emotional dispositions.*

GtK 7: Variations in Individual's Constitution: *Diurnal Effects*

*I*n the Lifestyle Medicine Series, we explored the idea of the biological clock in our body. In fact, many clocks are ticking in various parts of our body regulating the timely functioning of those organs, thereby creating a rhythm in the overall functioning of the body.

Similarly, in Ayurveda, there is a reference to the concept of the **Doshic Clock**, wherein the different doshas rise and fall in a cyclical fashion at different times during the day.

Some times of the day are characterized by dominance of one dosha over the others.

Different time periods have specific characteristics or qualities that influence the individual constitution.

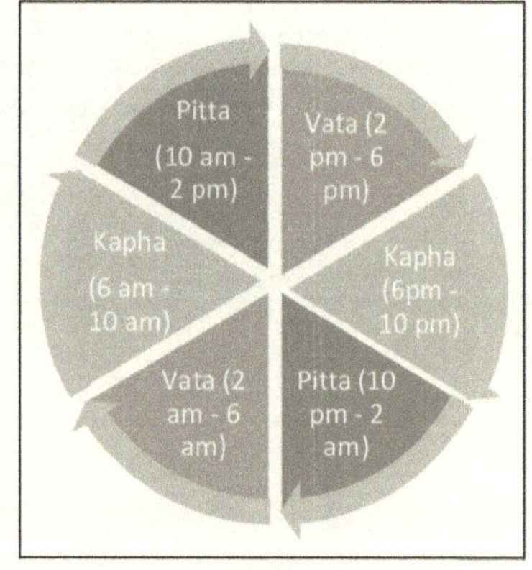

2:00 am – 6:00 am: This is the Vata period and is characterized by the clear, subtle, light properties of Vata dosha. Waking up in this time period influences our state of being with the qualities of Vata dosha and ensures a clear and active disposition to navigate through the day. Meditating early in the morning will help to regulate the same.

6:00 am – 10:00 am: This is the Kapha period and is characterized by the heavy and sluggish quality. Waking up in this time period gives rise to a heavier feeling in the body and mind. Because Kapha is cool and sluggish, the digestion will not be so great during this time. Hence breakfast is advised to be light.

10:00 am – 2:00 pm: This is the Pitta period and is characterized by the heat of the Pitta dosha, which aligns with the increasing heat of the external environment. Our digestive capacity, metabolic activity, and productivity are at a peak during this Pitta period. The largest meal of the day is advised in this period.

2:00 pm – 6:00 pm: This is again the Vata period, characterized by the transition from the day to the night. The qualities of Vata dosha remain dominant; creative activities find a place in this interval of time, as well as calming activities that keep the influences of Vata in balance.

6:00 pm – 10:00 pm: This is once again the Kapha period. Because of its influence, it is advised to have a light and an early dinner to ensure sufficient time for digestion. Going to bed at this period will help us fall asleep easily owing to the sluggish nature of the Kapha dosha.

10:00 pm – 2:00 am: This is the Pitta period. The body is active on the inside, setting up tasks of detoxification, cleansing, and rejuvenation. Remaining awake at this time will hamper these processes. Since Pitta kindles the fire of digestion, it stimulates hunger and upsets the normal rhythm.

How does this knowledge help?

Awareness of the Doshic clock helps us to plan our daily routine with particular reference to when to eat, how much to eat, when to sleep, etc. This will lead to a lifestyle that is energetic and productive while remaining healthy and well.

Practical Action

- *Take any one significant activity of your day. Observe the time period when you usually perform this activity. Study if the nature of the activity is in alignment with the doshic influence of that period. Note your observations.*
- *On the days when the alignment is missing, note the effects on your body and mind.*

12 GtK 8: Variations in Individual's Constitution: *Seasonal Effects*

Just as the changes occur in the nature of the dosha during the day, similar changes occur with the change in the seasons during the year. Ayurveda school recognizes this as an important influencer of health and wellbeing.

The nature of the season directly affects digestive capacity in an individual, resulting in either excess or poor digestion ability. This in turn influences the constitutional balance within the body and accordingly the energy or the strength of the person.

If the digestive capacity (or digestive fire *akin* to metabolism) is strong, the body can digest foods that are even heavier in nature. If the foods are lighter in quality, digestion and assimilation is faster resulting in tiredness or lack of energy within a short period after consumption.

Hence it is important to adapt food practices in line with our digestive ability.

If the fire is strong and the body does not get enough quantity and quality of foods in line with the strength of the fire, the fire then ends up absorbing the internal food stores. A similar phenomenon is observed in modern science, wherein during starvation, the internal food stores are used up by the body through specific metabolic processes[2].

---

[2] Refer to chapter for more details. *GtK 1:* Nutrition: *Energy, Metabolism, and Healthy Diet*

If the digestive fire is lacking, the food is not digested well which in turn results in the accumulation of toxins thereby affecting immunity.

Dynamically adapting food practices and other lifestyle changes with the changes in the environment will help the body to adapt to the seasonal changes.

As per the Ayurveda, the entire year is divided into six seasons or Ritus. The periods during the year may vary from region to region, but importance may be given to the nature and quality of season:

Winter or Shishira Ritu:

The weather remains cold and dry in this season.

There is an accumulation of Kapha dosha in the body. The digestive capacity is good.

Spring or Vasanta Ritu:

There is a gradual transition from the cold winter towards the warm Summer.

The onset of warmth in the environment melts the accumulated Kapha dosha and this is the time when Kapha related problems are observed. The digestive capacity tends to slow down.

Summer or Grishma Ritu:

The weather is characterized by intense heat and winds.

The previously vitiated Kapha tends to get pacified, while there is an accumulation of Vata dosha. The digestive capacity is mild.

Monsoon or Varsha Ritu:

The weather is characterized by clouds and rain.

The previously accumulated Vata dosha gets vitiated and now there is an accumulation of Pitta dosha. The digestive fire starts to enhance.

Autumn or Sharad Ritu:

The sky remains clear and the sunlight is bright.

The previously vitiated Vata dosha tends to pacify and the previously accumulated Pitta tends to further increase. The digestive capacity also increases further.

Late Autumn or Hemanta Ritu:

There is an onset of cold weather and cold winds.

The previously enhanced (vitiated) Pitta tends to get pacified. The digestive capacity is further enhanced.

How does this knowledge help?

Awareness of seasonal variations will help us adapt ourselves through lifestyle modification and avoid disturbance in our health and wellbeing. For example, during the winter, a Vata predominant person will aggravate the Vata in them more, if they continue to eat cold, raw salads (high in Vata) in the dry and cold of the winter.

Practical Action

- *Look at the current time of the year. Check what season it falls under. Observe the external environment and try to recognize the predominant dosha of the season.*
- *Observe your digestive strength and general energy levels. Correlate them with the nature of foods you eat.*

GtK 9: Variations in Individual's Constitution: *Age-Related Effects*

*T*he doshic predominance changes not only with the seasons and days but also with the age and growth of the individual. Different doshas take precedence in different ages and characterize the functioning and behavior of our bodies in that time period.

Childhood and Adolescence (Birth to 16 years of age)

- The **Kapha dosha** is maximum during this period of our life.
- These early years are characterized by growth, nourishment, and building up of strength.
- Common ailments experienced during these years will generally be Kapha related such as cold, cough, and allergies.

Adulthood and Middle-age (16 to 50 years of age)

- This period of our life is governed by the dominance of **Pitta dosha.**
- Exposure to a variety of activities and challenges in life, assimilation of information, and an increase in productivity, all relating to the Pitta dosha, characterize this period.
- The ailments generally experienced during these years will be Pitta related such as hyper-acidity and inflammations.

Elderly (50 years and above):

- The **Vata dosha** is most influential in this period of life.

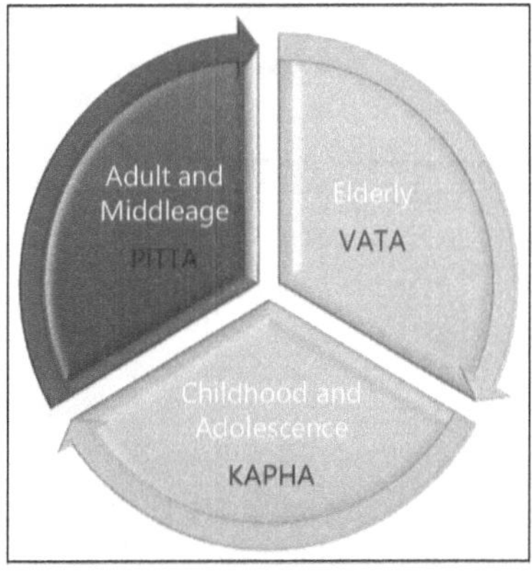

- The capacity of the body to rejuvenate on its own comes down and there is depletion in the overall energy levels. The needs of the body and mind become subtle and delicate, typical of the Vata characteristic.

- Ailments such as depression, dementia, joint pains, and insomnia are all typical of this phase of life and are Vata related.

How does this knowledge help?

This knowledge helps us to understand the changes in the body and mind with age and the need to dynamically adapt our lifestyles, and mental and physical activities accordingly. Not adapting our lifestyles can overburden our body and mind and disturb the health and harmony.

Practical Action

- *Take up any three individuals of different age categories in your close circle. Find out the doshic dominance specific to their age.*

- *Try to correlate their physical and mental disposition to the influence of the dosha governing their age. Note any five such correlations.*

14 GtK 10: Variations in Individual's Constitution: *Effects of Foods*

In the Ayurveda school of thought, foods and food practices assume high importance as part of daily routine. The constitutional balance is directly related to the ability of the body to digest what we consume and assimilate them into the system without overburdening the system. The digestive fire is influenced by the foods we eat. Similarly, the strength of the digestive fire that fluctuates with the external environment also influences the digestion and strength of an individual as we discussed in the previous chapter.

*To understand this, let us get familiar with two Ayurveda concepts and terms, particularly **Ojas and Digestive fire.***

At a physical level, the food that we eat after digestion is converted into basic elements that nourish the tissues. The finer essence or energy of these elements is called 'Ojas'. So Ojas is the end product of what we consume and can be either strong or weak depending on the quality of foods and our digestive ability.

If our Ojas is strong, our health, spirit (energy level), and immunity are strong. If our Ojas is weak, our energy and vitality become weak and will hamper our Immunity.

A good digestive fire results in the production of Ojas. However, weak digestion results in the formation of toxins (known as *Ama)*, which is the complete opposite of Ojas. The accumulation of Ama weakens Ojas and thereby reduces Immunity.

Let us now delve into the details of food types, their nature, and their qualities.

Ayurveda believes everything in the universe including the foods we eat is made up of five elements. The combination of elements gives rise to a **particular taste or Rasa** for that food. There are six types of Rasa recognized by Ayurveda.

Taste	Some examples	Predominant elements
Sweet	Rice, Wheat, Sugar, Milk	Earth + Water
Sour	Lemons, Tomatoes, Cheese	Earth + Fire
Salty	Rock salt, Sea salt, Celery	Water + Fire
Pungent	Onion, Garlic, Chillies, Pepper	Fire + Air
Bitter	Turmeric root, Coffee, Fenugreek (Methi)	Air + Ether
Astringent	Pomegranate, Unripe banana, Chickpeas	Air + Earth

Based on these elemental combinations we can relate their effects on the doshas of the body.

For example, we see that the bitter taste is made of the same elements as that of the Vata dosha. Hence, bitter foods tend to aggravate the Vata dosha. Similarly, the sweet taste is made up of the same elements as that of the Kapha dosha. Excess consumption will make the body prone to Kapha related diseases.

Taste	Effect on Vata	Effect on Pitta	Effect on Kapha	Taste
Sweet	Pacifies	Pacifies	Aggravates	Sweet
Sour	Pacifies	Aggravates	Pacifies	Sour
Salty	Pacifies	Aggravates	Aggravates	Salty
Pungent	Aggravates	Aggravates	Pacifies	Pungent
Bitter	Aggravates	Pacifies	Pacifies	Bitter
Astringent	Aggravates	Pacifies	Pacifies	Astringent

Foods are also classified based on their nature or quality as Satvik, Rajasik, and Tamasik.

While the physical constitution is based on Vata-Pitta-Kapha as discussed above, the subtler or mental constitution is influenced by the three qualities or Gunas of Nature, i.e. Sattva, Rajas, and Tamas.

Guna or Quality	State of Mind	Nature of foods	Examples of Foods
Satvik	clarity, lightness, and awareness.	Light and easy to digest. If eaten in adequate quantities, they build up Ojas and vitality.	Fruits such as Mango, Pomegranate, Coconut. Steamed vegetables, Sweet potato, Sprouts. Rice, Tapioca, Mung, Yellow lentils. Milk, fresh home-made yogurt, ghee, and cheese.

Guna or Quality	State of Mind	Nature of foods	Examples of Foods
Rajasik	activity, creativity, and passion.	Hot, spicy, and salty; stimulate senses. Excess of these foods excites and agitates the mind.	Sour fruits, Apples, Banana. Potato, Cauliflower, Spinach, Broccoli. Millets, Corn, Red Lentils. Spiced foods such as hot pickles, salted chips, Fish, Chicken.
Tamasik	inertia, lethargy, and heaviness.	Heavy and hard to digest. Excess of these foods will dull the mind and induce sleep and lethargy.	Avocado, Apricots, Plums. Mushrooms, Garlic, and Onions. Wheat and Brown rice. Dark meat, Beef, Lamb, Pork, Thick cheese. Old and stale foods also tend to be Tamasik.

How does this knowledge help?

- Food consumption is a vital activity. The food consumed will eventually become a part of us at the elemental level.
- Our food choices affect our health. Consider the scenario where a Kapha type of person continues to choose foods excess in Kapha that will eventually result in Kapha related disorders such as diabetes.

- Our food choices affect mental health as well. For example, excess of spicy or pungent taste results in anger, aggression, and envy, etc., all related to Pitta.
- Hence the knowledge of the body constitution, as well as that of the foods we consume, will enable us to maintain harmony within and thereby, our health and wellbeing.
- Note that no particular food is right or wrong; it is only the excess or reduction in particular food type (taste or quality) in the context of an individual's innate constitution that matters.

Practical Action

- *List the tastes of foods that you like and those that you dislike. Do you see the correlation between your constitution type and your preferences?*
- *Explore the qualities of the foods you eat and its effects on your mental state. Note them down.*
- *Make a few conscious adjustments of foods and observe their effects on your health, energy, and state of mind.*

15 GtK 11: More about Foods: *Practical Considerations*

Ayurveda believes that it is important to note what type of foods we eat, as that influences our constitution, as we discussed in the previous article. Furthermore, it suggests that how we process and consume foods also has implications on health and wellbeing.

Food and Constitution

- It is good to eat foods that are compatible with our constitution. For example, if our constitution type is Pitta, it is best to have fermented foods and spicy foods in moderation as the sourness would aggravate the Pitta further.
- It is also good to eat foods considering the changes in the constitution of the body due to changes in times and seasons. For example, in the hot and dry summer season, it is good to choose foods that reduce heat such as buttermilk and cucumber. Also, it is a good idea to have light and easily digestible foods in summer such as kichadi (lentil/ rice porridge) when the digestive capacity is relatively weaker in summer.
- Foods that are antagonistic in nature are to be avoided. There are food combinations specified in the Ayurveda classics that do not go well together. Example: Fish and Milk or Melons and milk, etc. which cause disturbances in the constitution.

Food and State of Mind

- Eat in a congenial place with due regard to hygiene and crowding, so that the mind is pleasant during the process.
- Enjoy the food with total concentration, so you are aware and conscious of how much you eat and how you eat.
- Eat in a relaxed and calm state.

Even though we eat the prescribed diet and in the right quantity, the food fails to get digested properly if eaten in an emotionally disturbed state such as in a rush or anxiety or grief, the moods alter the constitution and digestion.

Food and Discipline: *Few Dos and Don'ts*

- Eat at the right time of the day.
- Eat when hungry. Eat as much as that satisfies your hunger.
- Make sure you feel light after you eat. Overeating will lead to some distress or discomfort that indicates heaviness due to overconsumption.
- Do not eat when not hungry.
- Do not eat again soon after a meal.
- Do not eat hurriedly or too slowly.
- Do not eat foods that you cannot digest.
- Do not eat when constipated.
- Do not drink cold or chilled water, especially during the meal.
- Do not drink too much water or no water at all during a meal.
- Do not eat preserved and stale food.
- Do not eat frozen food.
- Do not eat too spicy, sour, or salty food.

How does this knowledge help?

- Types of foods as well as the manner of eating affects the constitution and thereby health and wellbeing.
- Remembering the pointers regarding food will make us aware of our current eating habits and observe their effects.

Practical Action

1. *Observe and make a note of the current eating practices you have. Also, make notes of how you feel after eating your meal (light or heavy). List some common health disturbances that you regularly feel (gastritis, fullness, heartburn, etc.)*
2. *Start with a few changes and observe how they impact your health and wellbeing.*

16 GtK 12: Immunity and Resistance: *Concepts in Ayurveda*

The ability of the body to protect itself against any disease-causing agent, and maintain good health is called the Immunity of the body. In Ayurveda, it is known as *Vyadhi Kshamatwa* [Vyadhi – disease; Kshamatwa- the ability to resist].

Immunity and Constitution

The physical and physiological strength (Immunity) of our body is considerably dependent on the doshic make up of our original constitution (*Prakriti*). Of the three doshas, Kapha dosha contributes most to the strength, stability, and Immunity of our body. Hence a Kapha dominant person has better strength and Immunity than other doshic types. However, the following factors are also vital and critical in deciding the strength of our Immunity:

- The foods we eat
- Our digestive capacity
- Our mental disposition
- Our conduct and behavior
- *In general, our lifestyle itself*

In the previous article, we explored the direct relationship between foods and Immunity.

The food that we eat is digested and converted into elements that nourish the tissues, the essence or energy of which is called '*Ojas*'.

If the resulting Ojas is strong, our health, spirit, and immunity are strong. If our Ojas is weak, our energy and vitality become weak, which hamper Immunity.

It is the *Agni* or the digestive fire that transforms foods into Ojas. A good digestive fire results in the production of strong Ojas. Similarly, weak digestion results in the formation of toxins or *Ama*. The accumulation of Ama weakens Ojas and thereby reduces Immunity.

Ways to Enhance Immunity

- Consume more fresh vegetables and fruits, whole grains, legumes, and dairy products. These get digested easily and make way for the production of Ojas.
- Eat according to the seasonal requirements. For example, eating raw, cold salads may not be suitable for all seasons. In winter, these raw, cold salads increase the dryness and cold property of the body, aggravating the Vata dosha. On the contrary, we have to opt for something hot, cooked, and nourishing.
- Cook the food well. It makes the food easy to digest and kills the germs.
- Consume freshly cooked and hot foods. It should be soft and easy to chew but not mushy.
- Add immunity boosting spices to the food. They not only enhance the taste and flavor but also make the food easily digestible.
- Different spices have different immunity boosting effects. For example, Jeera and Ajwain increase the digestive capacity and balance Vata and Pitta doshas in the body.

Turmeric has antiviral and antimicrobial properties. Black pepper and Mustard clear the channels for Ojas to reach the deeper tissues.

- Eat at a proper time. The main meal is best eaten in the middle of the day when the sun is at the highest and the digestion strongest. Eating a lighter meal for breakfast and at night, when digestion is relatively weaker would be better.
- Eat only to ¾th of one's capacity. Digestive fire is suppressed when one overeats. Overeating creates discomfort and the production of Ama. Eating the right amount for our body type enhances Ojas.
- Sipping lukewarm or room temperature water during the meal makes the food softer and easy to digest.
- Ghee is the easily digested fat – it contains essential fatty acids and is an immunity booster.

Things to be Avoided:

- Canned and processed foods are not advisable as they can be stale and hard to digest, denatured by processing, and may include chemical preservatives.
- Food starts to lose its potency after a few hours of cooking. It is better to avoid the preparation of a large quantity of food, and then refrigerating and reheating it. This makes food hard to digest; such foods result in Ama.

How does this knowledge help?

Ayurveda lays much emphasis on the prevention of diseases, and health promotion and Immunity is central to this. The knowledge as to how the lifestyle and food practices either increase or decrease Immunity is important to achieve optimal health and wellbeing.

The standard of practice in modern medicine to strengthen Immunity lays emphasis on nutrition and micronutrients in addition to exercises and other aspects. When this is complemented by the Ayurvedic school of thought that customizes recommendations to each individual, they both complement and go a long way in enhancing health and wellbeing.

Practical Action

1. *Make a note of your current status of Immunity in your own words: strong, moderate, or weak and why. Is there any correlation with some of the concepts you just read?*
2. *Of the pointers mentioned under "Ways to enhance Immunity", observe and note down how many you have been following. Also, note down what other pointers can be added to your list to be followed.*
3. *In a given week make a note of how many times you are using canned or processed food such as noodles, instant mixes, and the like.*
4. *Start with a few changes and observe how it impacts your health and wellbeing.*

GtK 13: Detox and Cleansing of The Body: *Five Ayurveda Practices*

Ayurveda recognizes that it is impossible to live a life without accumulating toxins and hence recommends procedures to remove the toxins out of the body. Five major procedures to remove the toxins from the body are indicated; they are popularly called *Panchakarma.*

Pancha means five and *karma* means action or practice in Sanskrit.

Panchakarma is administered both therapeutically as well as a preventative practice. Panchakarma practices are administered by Ayurveda physicians directly or by trained assistants under the supervision of a physician.

Panchakarma Phases and Techniques

There are three phases involved in administering the Panchakarma techniques.

Phase 1 is the preparatory procedure, known as *Poorva-karma* (Poorva means preparatory). This involves appetite enhancement, use of medicated oils (olcation), and sudation (sweating).

Phase 2 involves the main therapy or *Pradhana-karma* (Pradhana means main or important). This could be one of the following depending on the particular health needs.

Vamana (Emesis): This involves inducing vomiting therapeutically, to remove the excess of Kapha so as to have a clear, congestion-free chest. This is indicated in severe bronchitis, cold, cough, asthma, etc.

Virechana (Purgation): This involves the administration of therapeutic purgatives to eliminate the excess of Pitta. Disorders caused by the excess of Pitta such as skin rashes, inflammations, fever, nausea, and jaundice can be addressed by this therapy.

Basti (Enema): This involves administering medication rectally to remove the excess of Vata. Vata imbalance is a major cause for many disorders in the body and hence this is very useful to keep the Vata in balance.

Nasya (Nasal drops): This involves administering medication through the nasal passages in order to cleanse the excess of doshas in the throat, nose, sinus, and head areas. It is recommended to correct Pranic energy related disorders, migraine headaches, and certain eye and ear problems.

Rakta mokshana (Blood-letting): The toxins in the blood are purified by this therapy. It is used to treat conditions related to blood toxicity such as rashes, eczema, herpes, etc.

Phase 3 refers to post-therapy care or *Paschat-karma*. This includes rejuvenation and reviving of the digestive fire through appropriate food and lifestyle practices.

Benefits of Panchakarma

- Removes the root cause of diseases.
- Balances the Vata, Pitta, and Kapha doshas.
- Boosts immune system.
- Remove disease causing toxins.
- Increases physical and mental efficiency.

- Improves skin complexion.
- Helps in shedding extra weight.
- Helps alleviate insomnia, anxiety, and mental problem.
- Increases vigor and stamina.
- Increases the flexibility of joints.

How does this knowledge help?

Following these time tested practices and procedures to cleanse the body can help rejuvenate and revitalize the body.

If the disease or discomfort is too bothersome, one should meet the Ayurveda physician and plan a specific therapeutic option.

Even if one is healthy and fit, an appropriate Panchakarma option at regular intervals can be a good preventive or health promotion method, especially during the change in the seasons when the body needs the utmost support.

Practical Action

1. *Observe your current health status. Is there any health issue that has been consistently bothering and how does it relate to the excess of any particular dosha?*
2. *Which of the Panchakarma procedures may possibly help you?*
3. *Identify an Ayurveda physician nearby and seek an appointment for further analysis and planning or appropriate Panchakarma procedure.*

18 GtK 14: Oil Massage (Abhyanga): *Benefits and Process*

Abhyanga or massage with specific oils helps to nourish the body and has body strengthening and healing properties. Ayurveda recommends this as a regular practice, daily or weekly.

Specific oils are warmed and used for massaging and are advised as per the individual constitution. In addition to oils, ghee, herbal powders, and pastes are also used.

It can be done with simple oils at home as self-care at frequent intervals, or occasionally with medicated oils or herbal paste at Panchakarma centers.

Benefits of Abhyanga

Performing a self-care oil massage at least twice or thrice a week, will have numerous benefits for our body. They help to:

- Moisturize the skin
- Improve the blood circulation
- Calm the nerves system
- Rejuvenate the body and mind
- Improve the vision and reduce eye strain
- Provide relief from pain, headache, migraine, stress, and insomnia
- Relax muscles and reduce stiffness

- Prevent premature greying of hair, hair-fall, and dandruff
- Pacify Vata to prevent degenerative diseases

Process of Oil Massage: *Where and When?*

The best time is after light exercise and before shower while allowing 20-30 minutes between oil massage and shower.

However, in winter, it is done after the shower to mitigate the effects of excess Vata during the season.

Massage to the different portions of the body will help to pacify different doshas. Massaging the lower part of the body helps pacify Vata, the middle part pacifies Pitta and the upper part pacifies Kapha.

Massaging the scalp and foot regulates the movement of doshas throughout the body.

It is good to use locally available, cold-pressed oils for doing Abhyanga. Specific oils are recommended for the specific constitution.

Constitution type	Oils recommended
Vata	Gingelly oil, Jojoba oil, Almond oil, Castor oil
Pitta	Coconut oil, Sandalwood oil, Sunflower oil
Kapha	Castor oil, Mustard oil

Self-massage

Warm the oil by keeping the bowl of oil in hot water. Avoid directly heating the oil.

When massaging, give long strokes on long bones such as the arms and legs. Do this in one direction, always away from the heart.

Give circular strokes on joints like knees and elbows.

Use just the fingertips to apply oil and give small circular strokes to the scalp.

Practical Action

1. *Start with simple steps. Head massage or the body massage with the oil that suits your constitution. Document how you feel in the body and mind.*
2. *Start with once a fortnight and slowly take it to weekly or biweekly intervals.*
3. *Explore how this affects your energy and wellbeing during the day.*

2.3 Good to Know (GtK): *Yoga Series*

19 GtK 15: Yoga: *Concept of Disease and Health*

The science of Yoga believes that health and wellbeing is not a discrete state, rather a dynamic continuum. At one extreme exists what we refer to as death and at the other extreme, immortality. In between, there are numerous states of health, wellbeing, and sickness.

Five Koshas

Yoga recognizes that a human being exists in five dimensions or in other words, humans are made of five coverings (*koshas*). These include physical or food-sheath (Annamaya-kosha) as the outermost covering, Energy sheath (Pranamaya-kosha), Mind (Manomaya-kosha), Intellectual (Vignanamaya-kosha) in the middle, and Bliss (Anandamaya-kosha) as the innermost covering.

In the Anandamaya-kosha, a person enjoys harmony, has a balance of all faculties, one-mindedness, and is the healthiest. In the Vignanamaya-kosha, there arises discriminative ability of right and wrong. This influences the thought pattern in the Manomaya-kosha which is also regarded as the plane of origin of disease (*Vyadhi*). This then reflects changes in the Pranamaya-kosha and then the Annamaya-Kosha where the disease finally manifests as symptoms.

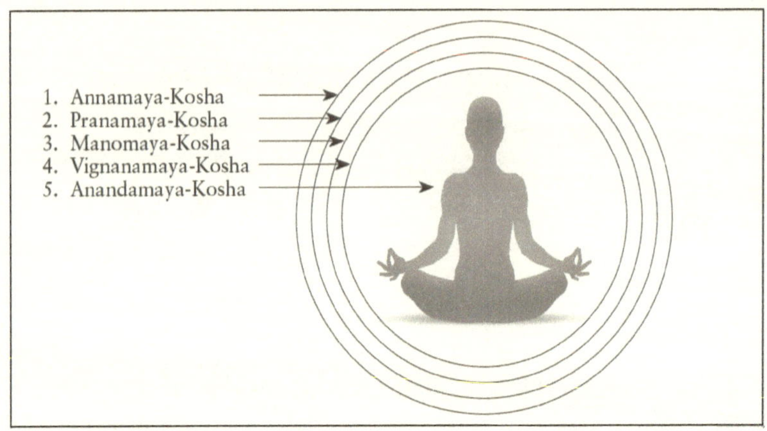

Optimal Health and Disease

Patanjali's Yoga philosophy defines optimal health as a state of mind that is peaceful, aware, and relaxed. Here there is a cessation of all deviations or modifications of the mind in the field of consciousness (*Chitta Vritti Nirodah*).

The field of Yogic Psychology is attracting huge attention in the recent years where mental health issues as well as psychosomatic disorders are on a rise.

Yoga also aligns with the Ayurvedic concept of disease as a state that is subject to disturbances in the harmony of the doshas (humors), dhatus (support structures of the human body), and rasas (fluids). Here too, the food habits (*Ahara*) and lifestyle (*Vihara*) assume high importance in keeping one healthy.

Yoga recognizes health and disease through specific traits and characteristics as illustrated below:

Attribute	Health	Disease
Body	Strong, no disease symptoms	Weak, disease symptoms such as fever, tremors, etc. can occur
Breath	Vital and energetic	Fast and weak

Attribute	Health	Disease
Mind	At peace	Restless
Attitudes	Positive	Negative orientation, pessimistic
Emotions	Moderate, healthy expression	Disturbed and volatile

Yoga for Holistic Development

Yoga aims to achieve the overall development of the human body-mind-self in an integrated way. Sage Patanjali first described and codified the Yogic knowledge into an eight-step (Ashtanga) philosophy and practice. The first two limbs, *Yama* and *Niyama* provide the code of conduct and discipline for character and value formation; *Asanas* help in strengthening of the body and mental discipline; *Pranayama* regulates the breath and the vital Prana; *Prathyahara* helps withdraw the senses and the mind inward toward the Self; *Dharana* stabilizes the attention on the high Self within; *Dhyana* helps to achieve a meditative state and connection with the inner Self; *Samadhi* represents a state of unity or one-ness with the inner Self.

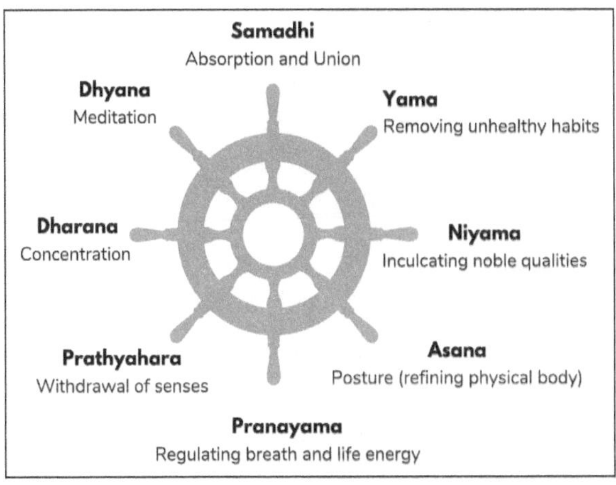

GtK 16: Yoga and Ayurveda: *Customized Yoga for Individuals*

Yoga and Ayurveda are closely related and complement each other. The final goal of Yoga is Self-realization. The goal of Ayurveda is to enhance the health and longevity of life. This is in view of preserving one's health until the goal of Self-realization is achieved.

Commonalities Between Yoga and Ayurveda

Yoga and Ayurveda originated around the same time. They have roots in a common philosophical thought that aims at the highest level of wellbeing for mankind.

Both Yoga and Ayurveda see the human being from a holistic point of view - made up of body, senses, mind, and spirit.

Both Yoga and Ayurveda use the same principles such as the theory of Pancha-bhutas (five elements) and Pancha-koshas (five bodies), doshic constitution of the body, etc.

How Yoga Finds a Place in Ayurveda?

The regimen prescribed by Ayurveda for the molding of mental makeup and personality is based on the Yamas and Niyamas (dos and don'ts) of the Yoga sutras.

Ayurveda recommends Yoga postures or Asanas particular to the individual body constitution to produce maximum health benefits for the Yoga practitioner.

Pranayama or breathing exercises as well as Dhyana or Meditation practice are prescribed in Ayurveda for the upkeep of mental health and balance of mind.

Yoga Based on Ayurveda Constitution

As we discussed earlier, Ayurveda believes that each individual is unique and provides personalized recommendations for lifestyle and food practices based on the constitution of the individual.

The same applies to Yoga postures and breathing exercises too. Different Yoga practices have different physiological effects on the body and they have to align with the constitutional makeup. And with the seasonal changes, Yoga practices need to be dynamically adapted rather than following a fixed regimen all through the year.

The variations are suggested in the type of asana, frequency, pace, and duration.

Few examples of Asanas specific to a Constitution:

For *Vata* type - *Sukhasana* (Easy posture), *Siddhasana* (Ready posture), *Padmasana* (Lotus pose)

For *Pitta* type - *Bhujangasana* (Cobra pose), *Sarvangasana* (Shoulder stand), *Halasana* (Plough pose)

For *Kapha* type - *Veerabhadrasana* (Warrior pose), *Dhanurasana* (Bow pose), *Vasisthasana* (Side plank pose)

Practical Action

1. *Try to include one or two simple asanas and breathing practices specific to your constitution in your daily regimen if not already practicing.*
2. *Observe the effects these bring about in your energy levels in addition to strength and fitness.*
3. *Assess your constitution with the help of an Ayurveda expert and enlist the specific Yoga exercises appropriate for you.*

21

GtK 17: Yoga Asanas and Pranayama: *Physiology and Benefits*

The two limbs of Yoga i.e. Asana and Pranayama have gained unprecedented attention as a way of strengthening the body and the mind. Asanas (postures) and Pranayama (breathing exercises) have been researched and well-studied for their effects on human physiology and their impact on wellbeing.

Asana, derived from a Sanskrit term – 'seat', means 'pose' or 'posture'. It is the third step in Patanjali's Yoga tradition.

The Yoga postures are of many types – sitting, standing, forward bending, backward bending, twisting, inversion, and supine. Each of them has many subtypes for fulfilling a particular purpose. Traditionally, about 84 different types of asanas are described and they have taken different names and forms at different times.

According to the Yoga tradition, the asana should serve the body in achieving a state of steadiness, stability, and happiness.

Pranayama or breath regulation forms the fourth limb of Patanjali's Yoga tradition and philosophy. Eight different types of Pranayama are suggested.

The breath is presumed to be connected both to the physical and the energetic body and thus it's regulation helps in achieving the harmony between the two.

The regulation of the energy or the Prana is the essence of inner wellbeing and health.

Physiologic Effects and Health Benefits

Yoga has a downregulating effect on Hypothalamic-Pituitary-Adrenal (HPA) axis and the sympathetic nervous system[3] thereby impacting various body systems – cardiovascular and respiratory, neuro-endocrine, digestion, metabolism, Immunity, etc. Specifically, the following effects are documented:

- *Decrease levels of cortisol and adrenaline*
- *Increase insulin sensitivity and reduce blood glucose*
- *Reduction of serum cholesterol*
- *Reduce heart rate and blood pressure*
- *Improve lung capacity*
- *Changes in brain waves (EEG - electroencephalogram) to the lower frequency (calmer) states*

Many studies have demonstrated the role of Yoga in complementing conventional treatments for several medical disorders. In some cases, long term Yoga has led to a reduction in the dosage of medications as well. The following health benefits are recorded in literature:

- *Physical fitness due to cardio-respiratory efficiency*
- *Hypertension and Coronary Atherosclerosis, protection against strokes and heart attacks*
- *Obesity and Diabetes*
- *Stress, Anxiety, and Depression*
- *Improved wellbeing and quality of life in cancer patients*

In a study among pregnant women, Yoga resulted in reduced stress and improved birth outcomes.

---

[3] For more details, refer to the chapter - GtK 5: Stress and Healthy Behaviors: The Neuro-physiology and its implications.

Note:

- While studies have documented the benefits of Yoga, it is also important to recognize that not all studies are controlled, randomized studies. The evidence ranges from strong to moderate.
- While Yoga has proven to play a complementary role, the patients are advised to comply with the conventional treatments and keep the treating physician informed of any lifestyle change.
- Yoga should be learned from a qualified Yoga trainer and preferably a Yoga therapist.

Practical Action

1. *If you have not started Yoga already, make a start. Find a good Yoga trainer and start with a few basic asanas and pranayamas.*
2. *Practice for a while and explore how it impacts your fitness and energy levels.*
3. *Also, get your constitution assessed by an Ayurveda physician and alter your Yoga practice for your constitution.*
4. *Document the difference in your strength, fitness, and energy levels.*

2.4 Good to Know (GtK): Meditation (Heartfulness) Series

22 GtK 18: Meditation on the Heart: *Philosophy and Practice*

Meditation is a time tested practice recommended by all religions and spiritual traditions. In the last few decades, the scientific exploration of the effects of Meditation on health and wellbeing is increasing.

There are many systems of Meditation today and they differ from one another, mainly in the process, the object, and the goals that they offer.

One who is interested in learning Meditation has to explore options with an open mind, choose a practice that offers clear goals and objectives, give a fair trial and test the system to assess its impact, and also study if a particular system is compatible to one's lifestyle.

Scientific literature helps a great deal, as well as the philosophy and tradition of the system, in selecting a method.

Two systems of Meditation have become global movements today; Heartfulness and Mindfulness systems. Both have roots in time tested traditions, are well tested in the field of science and wellbeing, and are widely practiced today.

Mindfulness practices help the individual to be mindful and achieve self-awareness.

Heartfulness practices also intend the same; in addition, they also help the practitioner in harnessing the deeper heart-based meditative conditions and consciousness.

In this series, we will cover the philosophy and practice of Heartfulness Meditation and supportive practices.

Meditation on the Heart: Philosophy of Heartfulness System

The Heartfulness system recognizes that the inner self or the heart is central to one's existence, just as the physiological heart is vital to the functioning of the body.

The individual who has lost connection with one's heart is deprived of peace, calm, and inner harmony. The mind is not in control, is distracted, and lacks focus. This is pronounced when the individual is subjected to various stressors in life, that may be internal or external. Such a mind falls short of its optimal performance and productivity. Stress can result in fears and anxieties that hamper health and wellbeing.

On the other hand, when the mind is regulated and centered on the heart, it calms down and becomes an effective instrument. The mind that continually stays centered on the heart becomes a channel for the heart's intelligence and qualities to express through the mind.

Not only the individual enjoys peace and harmony, but the performance improves too and so does one's wellbeing and quality of life.

With time, the heart's qualities such as love, compassion, balance, poise, harmony become the foundation of one's existence.

Heartfulness Practices

Heartfulness practice is also known as 'Sahaj Marg' or 'Natural Path' and it has been practiced in its current form for over 100 years. With roots in India, it is currently practiced by millions of practitioners in more than 160 countries.

The system is a simplified and modified form of Patanjali's Raja Yoga to suit the needs of the current times. The training is offered to people from all walks of life and backgrounds, through a system of volunteers who are certified Meditation trainers.

They help to start Meditation with initial few training sessions followed by personal coaching and follow up support. The training and coaching services are provided for life and are free of charge, with a vision of making the world a better place, a place where the heart and mind are connected and in harmony.

Four basic practices are offered to those who are interested in the beginning. These have guided techniques that are well researched, simple, and practical. They include:

- *Heartfulness Relaxation*
- *Heartfulness Meditation*
- *Heartfulness Cleaning*
- *Heartfulness Prayer*

The guided techniques can be found as annexures at the end. The audio and video versions are available on the website.

The relaxation technique helps to relax the body and mind and is a pre-requisite for Meditation.

Meditation practice uses self-suggestions to bring the attention to the heart and allow it to rest there passively. Thoughts that occur are allowed to pass on; they are simply to be ignored so the attention comes back to the heart.

The effects of Meditation are observable and experienced in the first few sessions in the form of relaxation, calm, peace, joy, etc.

With regular practice, over a period of time, one can experience deeper and profound changes. Meditation is suggested in the morning so the mind is well prepared to navigate through the day in a state of calm and poise. The other two techniques: cleaning and prayer will be discussed in the next chapter.

Relevance of Meditation in Lifestyle Change

Our lifestyle and habits have roots in our thoughts, beliefs, and the choices we make. A regulated and calm mind is discriminative and can make the right choices.

A heart centric mind will not lose sight of the larger vision and hence can better manage the distractions that we face in our daily lives.

Over time, the beliefs and behaviors change and this will reflect on the health and wellbeing.

In the last chapter, we will discuss the benefits of Meditation from a scientific perspective.

Practical Action

1. *Try the Heartfulness relaxation and Meditation and document the changes before and after the Meditation.*
2. *Fix up 20 minutes of your time in the morning for Meditation and try for one week. Document what impact it has on your thoughts and actions.*
3. *Contact a nearby certified trainer[4] for your personal coaching and follow up support. Download the heartsapp[5] and access online support.*

---

[4] https://heartspots.heartfulness.org/
[5] https://heartsapp.org/

GtK 19: Decluttering the Mind: *Process and Effects*

In the last chapter, we discussed Heartfulness Meditation as a tool to center oneself. A common experience that everyone encounters during meditation is the disturbing nature of thoughts that wouldn't allow one to dive deep into one's heart.

One realizes that these thoughts are because of the clutter that we pick up during our day to day activities and interactions.

How do we declutter our minds so that we can enjoy good Meditation? Heartfulness offers a cleaning technique for this purpose.

Heartfulness Cleaning

The philosophy of the Heartfulness system suggests that our minds gather impressions during its course of activities during the day. Whether we are at work or on a holiday, when the minds are engaged actively and emotionally, we gather the impressions that settle in the subconscious. Psychology also reaffirms this phenomenon.

These impressions then become the seeds for our thoughts and actions. Some impressions that are strong and deep-rooted transform into our tendencies and later form the basis of our personality. Hence we see such diversity and variations in activities and behaviors of people.

Heartfulness cleaning aids removal of impressions and slowly bring about the change in our thoughts and tendencies.

Heartfulness cleaning is done in the evenings after the completion of activities for the day. This is a self-guided mental process that uses suggestions to remove the impressions from the mind.

The mind's natural and original state is a state of purity and simplicity. The practice of cleaning restores this state at the end of the day.

This particular state helps in many ways: restores the connection with one's heart, helps to better manage work and family lives, prepares one for a good night's sleep. Some research findings in this space will be discussed in the next chapter.

Heartfulness Prayer

There is yet another technique that Heartfulness offers – Prayer, also referred to as a tool to connect with one's inner self.

This technique is used just before going to bed, as the last activity. This process involves recollection of the day's events and one's handling of them, the emotional highs and lows, and then resolving and visualizing a better version of oneself for tomorrow.

This is followed by the self-guided prayer to dive deeper into oneself. This prepares one for a deeper sleep and for the morning Meditation.

Jointly, all the four practices complement each other and help one's mind stay calm and in harmony all through the day and night.

The guided techniques can be found as annexures. The audio and video versions are available on the website.

Relevance to Lifestyle Change

A lifestyle change is a complex process that involves the body, mind, and heart. Cleaning removes the barriers that impede change. Particularly when complexities and impurities or the clutter in the head is removed, the choices and behaviors are more appropriate for one's wellbeing.

A heart-centric mind is also strong willed and helps to sustain lifestyle changes without effort.

The cleaning and the prayer directly impact sleep quality, thereby impacting Immunity and wellbeing.

Practical Action

1. *Try the Heartfulness cleaning and document the changes in your body-mind before and after the cleaning.*
2. *Try the Heartfulness prayer before going to sleep and assess its impact on sleep quality.*
3. *Fix up 20 minutes of your time in the evening for cleaning, and five minutes for prayer. Try this for one week. Document what impact it has on your emotions and behaviors.*
4. *Contact a nearby certified trainer[6] for your personal coaching and follow up support. Download the heartsapp[7] and access online support.*

---

[6] https://heartspots.heartfulness.org/
[7] https://heartsapp.org/

24   GtK 20: Heart-Centric Meditative Lifestyle: *Science and Implications*

Previously we learned about four practices that Heartfulness offers to help us connect our minds to the heart and achieve inner harmony and balance. All the four practices complement each other and help an aspirant to adopt a way of life that is Heart-centric.

'Heart-centric meditative lifestyle', also called 'Living Heartfully', has many implications on health and wellbeing that we will discuss in this chapter.

Let us first explore what 'Living Heartfully' actually means. This has been a topic of philosophical thought and debate for a long time and in recent times, it has attracted considerable attention from the scientific community too.

From a philosophical standpoint, the heart is regarded as the seat of one's true nature or character. A person is identified by one's heart either as a warm-hearted or a stone-hearted person. The feelings that arise in the heart fuel the thoughts and actions. Openness in one's heart and mind is what helps someone learn and evolve.

In any walk of life or endeavor, be it one's study or a career or a relationship, one has to apply one's heart fully into it to be successful. The heart is also regarded as the seat of divinity, one's inner self, or the soul, and hence offers the best or the highest potential that can be harnessed.

Scientific Studies Related to Heartfulness Practices

Heartfulness Meditation research studies have documented a reduction in stress levels and burnout, improvement in emotional wellness among the doctors and nurses working in a health facility in the U.S. in a span of 12 weeks interval.

Similar findings are reported by those who have participated in corporate wellness programs.

The same study in the U.S. also reported an increase in telomere length, particularly among the younger subjects.

Telomeres are cap-like structures on the chromosomes and their length indicates longevity in the life of the cells. Stress is shown to result in wear and tear of telomeres and hence the current study shows that Heartfulness practices seem to have protected the subjects from stress induced telomere damage.

A study by the National Institute of Mental Health and Neurosciences (NIMHANS) in India reported higher levels of wellbeing, positivity, satisfaction, lower levels of negative feelings, and lower perception of stress among long term Heartfulness practitioners.

The NIMHANS study also reported calmer and deeply relaxed states as measured by alpha, delta, and theta waves in both long term and short term Meditation practitioners indicating that Meditation can result in relaxed states quite early in the practice. The electroencephalogram (EEG) picked up few other characteristic findings such as Occipital Gamma waves (in the back of the brains) in long term meditators which indicate heightened perception, vision and expanded consciousness. The discussions of these findings are outside the scope of this chapter, and are described in detail in a manuscript that is published in a reputed journal.

Another study in the U.S. among chronic insomnia (sleeplessness) patients revealed improvement in sleep quality and duration over eight weeks.

Here Heartfulness practices (Relaxation, Meditation, Rejuvenation) and sleep hygiene were part of the intervention in addition to the routine sleep medication. The sleep quality as measured by what is called insomnia index doubled over 8 weeks (mean score reduced from 20 to 10) and over 85% of patients were withdrawn of the medication.

The authors discussed that Heartfulness practices led to higher levels of calmness, relaxation, acceptance, and confidence that eventually led to the changes.

Another study in India by a team of cardiologists showed that Heartfulness practices can regulate the autonomic nervous system (ANS). ANS modulation impacts both physical and psychological wellbeing[8].

The study showed a reduction in heart rate variability (HRV), blood pressure, and heart rate. The subjects also reported an increase in levels of peace and happiness as measured by the standard scales.

Scientific research continues to shed light on how Heartfulness Meditation practices impact physiology and psychology, thereby contributing to health and wellbeing.

Healthy Communities for Healthy World

In addition to the changes described above, there are many other changes related to communication, behavioral and managerial traits, areas that are not yet scientifically explored.

---

[8] For more details, refer to chapter GtK 5: Stress and Immunity: Effects, Physiology, and Healthy Behaviors

We will discuss these within the philosophical framework of the Heartfulness system.

In the last few years, the Heartfulness outreach activities have been stepped up to meet the growing needs to enhance mental health and wellbeing, performance within the office spaces, corporates, health and hospitality sector, universities, schools, and community spaces across the world.

Millions of new aspirants have reported anecdotally, the changes they felt in their body, mind, and heart. Slowing down of thoughts, relaxation, lightness, calmness, peace, and harmony, etc.

Heartfulness attributes these effects to its unique practice fueled by a very subtle energy called 'Yogic Transmission' that is practically and experientially verifiable by the practitioners. The Heartfulness teams encourage new aspirants to incorporate Heartfulness as part of their lifestyle so that these changes can be pronounced and sustained.

As reported by the long term practitioners, these practices have the potential to transform their personalities into becoming beings that are permanently calm, relaxed, and balanced.

Improved focus, work-family life harmony, refined and perceptive communication that translate into richer relationships both within families and workspace, enhanced productivity and efficiency, and many other results are an outcome of a Heart-centric meditative lifestyle.

Recognizing the need of the world today, the Heartfulness Institute offers focused programs on Heartful communication, Heart based leadership and management, Heartful relationships and parenting, etc.

The vision of the movement is to enable better alignment of the mind with the heart so the heart-based qualities of love, peace, and harmony may come forward in creating families, workspaces, and regions that are united and constructive.

A United World is the goal, knowing fully that there lies the wellbeing of mankind and their ecosystem.

Living Heartfully has many implications on health and wellbeing, not just for the individual or community, but for the planet and the whole ecosystem.

While science can measure some aspects of biological and psychological phenomena, there is much more that is not amenable for scientific research but available for experience. This needs verification and acceptance at a personal level.

The wellbeing of the individuals depends on the environment within the family or workspace and the community. Environment and other lifeforms are a part of the ecosystem and to address the issue at hand in a holistic manner, Heartfulness offers much promise through its practical and experiential tools and programs.

For more details, the reader is suggested additional reading of Heartfulness literature as listed in the references.

Practical Action

1. *Observe the impact of Heartfulness practice on your way of life: communication, reactions, relationships, and performance.*
2. *Make a self-assessment of how Heart-centric your life is at the moment and set a goal and a 90-day challenge to increase your Heart-centricity.*
3. *Observe the impact of the Heart-centric lifestyle on your overall wellbeing, family, and work life.*

25 GtK 21: Fasting and Silence: *Their Effects on Health and Wellbeing*

In the previous chapter, we referred to Heart-centric meditative lifestyle and we discussed its implications on several tenets of our life – communication and relationships, family and work life, etc. We also briefly reviewed some recent research findings as to how Heartfulness practices positively impact health and wellbeing.

In this chapter, we will briefly discuss two time-tested approaches that impact physical and mental wellbeing and are widely practiced across the globe by people from all walks of life and backgrounds. One of them 'Fasting' has attracted significant attention in the scientific world in recent years and the other one 'Silence' is yet to be explored.

There is no particular reason why this chapter is included in the Meditation series. The Heartfulness system does not mandate these practices but leaves it to the discretion of the practitioner to use them as additional tools at the time of need, in particular circumstances or training when greater focus and absorption is required on the part of the trainee.

However, in a broader religious, spiritual, and philosophical context – both 'fasting' and 'silence' have been offered as powerful tools for self-transformation. They particularly are suggested to remove the deeper tendencies and emotions which often become stumbling blocks to connect to the higher vision. The higher vision has been expressed in various forms: God or the Self or simply one's higher (real) nature.

Fasting

Let us begin with the current scientific understanding of the benefits of fasting.

The fasting state lowers insulin levels, burns the fat, and reduces weight[9]. Additionally, various lab studies have shown that fasting improves metabolism, lowers blood sugar, reduces inflammation, and has positive effects on allergic conditions such as arthritic pain and asthma, clears toxins, improves cognition, and reduces the risk of cancer.

Starvation can stimulate a physiologic process called **Autophagy** which means self-eating. This is a process that removes toxins, debris, and damaged cells in the body, and is part of self-preservation of the body. The cancer cells are removed through this process and hence cancer risk reduction is also one of the benefits discussed in the context of fasting.

Particularly intermittent fasting has been extensively studied. As against total fasting, intermittent fasting includes time-restricted eating where the food intake is confined to eight hours (between 7 am and 3 pm) or twelve hours (between 7 am and 7 pm).

This has shown to result in several health benefits: weight loss in obesity, prevention of diabetes and cancers, etc. Experts suggest that intermittent fasting should align with circadian rhythm, healthy diets, and lifestyle. Few studies have also reported an increase in stress resistance and longevity.

---

[9] For more details of fasting and insulin, refer to the chapters GtK 1 (Nutrition) and PIA 2 (Diabetes Mellitus)

Total fasting is found to be not sustainable as compared to intermittent fasting. Semi-fasting with liquids, fruits, and light foods is also practiced in several contexts.

In addition to the advantages mentioned above, fasting can also help to keep the body and mind light, and allows the body systems certain rest and rejuvenation.

Fasting can also bring discipline and self-restraint to overcome certain habits and behaviors that may be harmful to mental and physical wellbeing.

Silence

Few studies have documented health benefits of practicing silence as a practice.

Lowering of blood pressure and stress as a result of the lowering of cortisol and adrenaline;

neurogenesis in the hippocampus part of the brain that is associated with learning, memory, and emotions;

strengthen the immune system;

hormone regulation and prevention of plaque formation in arteries.

Periods of silence and pause from hectic lifestyle results in heightened self-awareness, reflections to connect the dots, big picture thinking, finding creative solutions to problems, etc. Hence, it can result in higher confidence and self-esteem.

Meditation results in the same effects by producing silence in the mental realm.

Heartfulness practices slow down the activity of mind and intellect and silence them on the surface; the heart that is the seat of feelings and creativity takes over and uses the mind as an instrument to solve the problems that otherwise seem complex.

Here the silence is not so much physical as much as it is a state or a condition that is established inside. This state of silence is practical and highly beneficial in the real world.

Yet from a lifestyle change perspective, incorporating 'fasting' and 'silence' for some time during the day or once a week, can be a great start.

It is important not to force this, but plan it in a self-sustainable way. It is important to look at these practices not in isolation, but as part of a larger lifestyle package.

Note: For those with health conditions like diabetes and eating disorders, they should consult their treating physician before planning any fasting procedure. Pregnant women and breastfeeding mothers should refrain from any type of fasting.

Practical Action

1. *Dedicate a day in a fortnight or a month and practice fasting and silence. Take any one at a time.*
2. *Observe the physical and mental changes as a result of the practice.*
3. *Document how it impacts on your health and wellbeing.*

2.5 Integrative Lifestyle Template

GtK 22: Integrative Health and Wellbeing Lifestyle: *A Template*

So far, we have covered theoretical details of several lifestyle components offered by Modern Medicine, Ayurveda, Yoga, and Meditation. At the end of each chapter, we have explored simple and practical ways of implementing them.

The highest gains in health and wellbeing can be experienced if all can be integrated together as part of one's lifestyle. How do we practically integrate them all? Where do I start?

This chapter provides a simple template to address these questions in the real world setting.

Fix First Things First

Fix in a Day

Start with simple basics when you begin to regulate your daily lifestyle. Fix those things that give you more than 50% headway.

In some mysterious way, you see that fixing things is actually fixing time.

It will not get any simpler than this. This chapter will provide you a list of things that you can fix as part of your routine. You can start fixing things either all at once or one after the other, depending on your comfort.

It is important that you bring this change as naturally as possible and at the same time you are able to enjoy this process.

- **Fix your time for waking up and going to bed.** *Through this, you have already begun to regulate your circadian rhythm which is a great start.*
- **Fix a time for your morning meditation, evening cleaning, and bedtime prayer.** *Now you are training your mind to be regulated and flexible, so the changes that you will introduce later will seamlessly become a part of your routine.*
- **Fix meal and snack time between 7:00 am and 7:00 pm.** *Remember the advantages of time-restricted intermittent fasting. This provides protection from a whole range of health issues that are prevalent today. For those who cannot complete the evening meal before 7:00 pm, try and keep at least two hours between your last meal and the sleep. Maintain at least 12 hours of fasting time after the last meal of the day is over, i.e. between your dinner and breakfast. Avoid any snack or even coffee in between. (However, intermittent fasting is not recommended for those who are diabetic and on medications or those who have any health issue, in which case one has to follow the treating physician's orders.)*
- **Fix your Yoga and exercise time in the morning.** *If you are starting for the first time, start off with 15 minutes Yoga and 15 minutes exercise and slowly take it to 30 minutes each. You don't have to do both together. You can distribute them between the morning and evening or even during the office hours while keeping a gap of a few hours between your meals and Yoga/exercise.*
- **Fix a time for short relaxing and rejuvenating breaks during working hours.** *Once every few hours, you can do a few minutes of deep breathing (alternate nostril or left nostril), do chair Yoga or some stretches, walk across the office and outside for fresh air, and a few minutes of meditation to*

reconnect with the heart. These pauses restore the inner connectivity and calm and help bring out creativity at the workplace as well as personal wellbeing.

- **Fix your family time, your personal relaxing and reading time in the evening.** *This helps to achieve fulfillment and contentment, which are important in the long run. In the evening hours, this prepares one for a good night's sleep.*

Note: *If your work extends into late hours or is erratic that does not begin and end at definite times, introduce short Meditation – relaxation – unwinding – fresh air walks – Yoga, and exercise times within your work-life.*

Fix in a Week

- **Fix a time for two days a week in the morning for a head massage with oil.** *Use the oil that suits your body constitution and the seasonal variations. Massage the scalp gently and give a time gap of 20 to 30 minutes before head bath.*
- **Fix a time for two days a week in the night for sole (feet) massage with oil.** *Use the oil that suits your body constitution and the seasonal variations. Apply the oil on your soles before going to bed.*
- **Fix one day in a week for total body massage with oil.** *You can do this as a weekend practice. Use the oil that suits your body constitution. If possible, expose your body to sunlight for some time. Give two hours and take bath.*
- **Fix a day in a week for a group and individual Meditation session with the local Heartfulness trainer.** *While daily practice helps to a certain extent, there are regular challenges and clarifications that can be addressed by a trainer. Participating in the weekly group sessions greatly enables the depth and grounding in the Heartful Meditation.*

Fix in a Year

- **Fix a day once a month or two for fasting.** *You can incorporate this on a weekend or on a holiday when you are free from your office work. Let your family know of the purpose so they can support you. If complete fasting is not possible, take liquids and fruits. (Fasting is not advised to diabetics or those who have any health issues.)*

- **Fix a day once a month or two for the practice of silence.** *You can incorporate this on a weekend or on a holiday when you are free from your office work. Let your family know of the purpose so they can support you.*

- **Fix a day or two every quarter for a Heartfulness retreat or a seminar.** *Heartfulness Institute offers seminars and retreats regularly that help an aspirant get deeply grounded in a heart-based way of life.*

- **Fix a day once every four months for total body detox and cleansing at a Panchakarma facility.** *Make sure the panchakarma procedure is advised and supervised by a trained Ayurveda physician who knows your constitution and specific requirements. Sometimes the procedures will change depending on the season, health, and other aspects.*

Note

- *Refer to the specific chapters for knowledge of 'what' and 'how' of a particular procedure or intervention.*

- *Initial contact with a lifestyle medicine physician or your family physician will help to understand specific advice on the diets, exercises, and habits.*

- *Connect with an Ayurveda physician to understand your unique constitution and plan your dietary regulation, daily routine, oil massage, and detox procedures.*

- *Learn Yoga specific to your requirements from a certified Yoga therapist or a trainer who works in collaboration with the Ayurveda physician. Stay connected to the Yoga trainer until you learn the practices and have integrated them into your routine.*
- *Stay connected with the nearby Heartfulness Meditation trainer for weekly follow-up support, group sessions, and retreats.*
- *Please refer to the template in the annexure for planning.*

SECTION 3

Making Lifestyle Change:
Inspired Action (IA) Series

27   IA 1: Have Vision and Goals for Health and Wellbeing

Our mind needs the motivation to change any aspect of our lives. When change is expected of something as complex as 'Lifestyle', motivation isn't enough. Now we have to find inspiration from within. Often we have experienced this: many a resolve on the new year eve wouldn't last for long. Resolutions made out of external motivation are a good start but need to be supported by inner inspiration to last long.

Making a resolve intellectually or emotionally will continue to need intellectual and emotional stimulation and hence the stimuli is still from external factors. When the stimuli disappear, the motivation dips.

Think of the changes that have lasted and have become a natural part of your life now and compare them with those that did not last. What could be the reason?

We all relate to having a 'Vision' for our education, career, or personal life. Often our health and wellbeing is not a part of the larger vision. In some way, we take it for granted, more so when we are busy chasing our career and other personal goals. *Is this your situation now? If so, this is the place to start.*

A vision to see oneself as a Health and Wellbeing champion enjoying high Quality of Life, and to become an inspiring force to others is the need of the hour.

A vision that is of a high order and complements visions in other departments of one's life is helpful and practical too. For example, Good health and wellbeing can only increase performance and efficiency and boost one's career. A fulfilling career impacts personal life too. It is important to see these linkages while envisioning the goals for oneself.

A high level of vision isn't enough.

It has to be broken up into smaller goals that are time bound, tangible, and achievable. This helps to stay motivated until we get to the end. Now imagine, what is it that helps us stay motivated throughout our lifetime because health and wellbeing will continue to need attention till the end. Such an inspiration that has to last for life must come from within, from the depths of the heart.

The next question is how do I find my vision and how do I stay connected with it, so it becomes a sustainable inspiration that lasts forever?

Here, the tools and practices such as meditation, contemplation, and journal writing provide help. Heartfulness Meditation and other supportive practices facilitate this in a natural and practical way. One may explore and experience it for oneself.

In the beginning, it appears like an intellectual or emotional exercise. The vision may appear as vague and non-realizable. It does not matter. Write down whatever comes. Revisit the same after a few days. It may appear as a more refined one. Write it down again till the vision appears clearly and you feel convinced from within.

At the same time, the vision should be tangible. Let us take an example.

Let us say my vision is to become an Integrative Health and Wellbeing champion. Now, who is a champion? We can define champion in our context as someone who manages to practice most of the components that we discussed in the template for an ideal lifestyle (previous section). I can set goals such as being able to practice 70% of the components in an year's time.

Practical Action

1. *Write down in your journal: what is your vision for life? And career?*
2. *After one of your Meditation sessions, give a thought to the vision for your wellbeing and health. What appears as your personal vision?*

IA 2: Maintain Your Personal Wellbeing Journal

In the previous chapter, we talked about setting vision and goals. Pursuing them in a systematic and disciplined way is the next step.

Many of us are resistant to the idea of a disciplined or structured lifestyle. Often, we give up even before we start based on our previous experience.

Let us explore if there is something we can learn from science in this regard.

In Nature, everything is systematic and rhythmic, be it the cycles of day and night, or the seasons. Human biology aligns its functioning with certain rhythm and order too. You may have come across the term 'Circadian Rhythm' or the 'Biological Clock'. Recent research shows that our body does not have one biological clock, rather every organ system has one, and they all work in harmony with each other. As far as we had aligned our waking-eating-sleeping pattern of lifestyle with the natural rhythm, we enjoyed optimal levels of health and wellbeing. In the last few decades, it is our lifestyle that has taken a beating and at the root of it is the disorderliness of our waking-eating-sleeping pattern. Many studies have shown how the changes in our sleep cycles and food habits have resulted in disorders that we experience today.

How to establish this structure in my lifestyle?

The scientific facts are compelling. I also have a vision and many small goals as stepping stones to achieve my larger vision. Here is where a personal wellbeing journal helps.

We can break our vision into small goals: yearly, six-monthly, 3-monthly, and monthly, and list them in a journal. These small goals are important so we start with easy ones, low hanging fruits as we say. Pick up a few that you can achieve with minimal effort and gain confidence and motivation. It doesn't matter what others do and how fast. This is a journey you need to walk and it is a personal one. You can decide the pace at which you would like to walk. And it is important that we get to the end.

What are the easy ones? Well, in many wellbeing champions' experience, waking up early in the day has not been an easy one to start off. It is probably a good idea to come to it later. Rather, 'say no junk food this week', or 'fix 10 minutes in the morning for daily meditation', or 'three cycles of sun-salutation Yoga every day', or 'three times of deep and slow breathing a few times during the day', can be the ones you may want to consider.

Let this list come out of your contemplation after a session of meditation or two. Decisions out of a mind that is calm and Heart-centred are inspired from within; they are also the ones that matter the most in a practical sense at any given time.

List a few that you want to take up for this month. It is preferable to take up at least one or two under each category of Integrative Health and Wellbeing Lifestyle:

- Lifestyle changes: Wake up time, sleep, habits, screen time, social media usage, etc.
- Food changes: Fixing time, quantity, and quality of foods.

- Yoga exercises.
- Breathing exercises and those specific to constitution or health status (you can list the one or two that you want to focus during the month and add one the others the next month).
- Meditation Practices: Techniques such as Heartfulness relaxation, Meditation, cleaning, connecting with the self, etc.
- Others: Any other that you think is relevant and does not fit under one of the above categories.

At the end of this hand-book, a '**Personal Wellbeing Journal Tracker**' format is provided as an annexure. You can take a print out of it and use it as a tool. Here, you can write down your vision and list the goals you want to achieve during the month. The tool helps you to keep track of what was achieved and what wasn't. It gives a snapshot of your monthly progress and also provides space to document what went well, what didn't, and why, so this learning can help you plan the next month.

Practical Action

1. *In order to get there, what are the low hanging fruits or smaller goals you have to accomplish?*
2. *What are some realistic and practical timelines for you?*

29 IA 3: Develop an Observer (Researcher) Mindset

So far, we have discussed Vision and Goals, and the importance of maintaining a personal wellbeing journal so we can start off well on our wellbeing journey. However, to stay on the course, we need the company of an observer who is objective and impartial and provides valuable guidance at every point in time. It is this guidance that brings us back on track every-time we take a detour. Especially with the lifestyle change, we are all aware of the distractions and temptations on the path. These can lure our intellect and emotions to convince and justify as right, whatever we may do. It is precisely here, the objective observer in me has to speak out, and for it to speak out loud and clear, I need to nurture it well.

But who is this observer? Is it a person or is it just my mind, or attitude?

It probably is everything about this. We are all familiar with the different voices within us, especially when we are caught up between two choices, and it is hard to zero down on one.

Take a moment to reflect: where do these two voices come from? What is the root of it? How is it that our mind speaks different voices?

In the fields of Yoga and psychology, this is very well studied. We also explored this in the Heartfulness philosophy in the previous section.

We exist at many levels – body, mind, and the deeper self. From within the mind, the intellect fueled by knowledge, and the emotion fueled by ego can pull us in different directions and often wouldn't let us think and act in the right direction. Hence, the mind regulation through meditation is so much emphasized in Yoga as this can help to eliminate the conflicting forces, resolve them, and bring them into unison. When the conflicts and confusion settle down, we are able to hear very clearly one voice from within. Having heard this, we now only have to act next.

Are there simple and effective techniques to address these conflicting forces?

Heartfulness Institute provides cleaning (decluttering the mind) technique precisely for this purpose. Supported by the cleaning technique, Meditation slowly strengthens the observer from within. It is worth exploring this and experiencing it directly.

The objective observer in oneself will need to be nurtured by us over time so it becomes a valuable and permanent guide on our onward journey. A good time to start the lifestyle change is when the motivation is high. Hence, it is important to make Meditation and cleaning, as part of a lifestyle change from the very beginning so the observer is nurtured and strengthened. It is like you are building a second-line leader whom you can then delegate your tasks to, and your effort and energy is less after a while. When you continue to nurture the observer, the deputy will then transform into a permanent valuable guide.

Hence, it can be rightly called a Researcher Mindset.

We all relate to how science and research bring facts into our lives and provide valuable direction. We trust that a good research is unbiased, and provides solutions for our wellbeing. In research too, there is a system of aggregation of results and will provide only what is good for the majority. Depending on the statistical methods adopted, the research may provide results that may be generalized to 90% or 95% of the population wherever the research study took place. Thus, even in a well-done research study, it is still a standard and general guidance for the population at large and may not necessarily apply to every individual.

While this applies well to treatments and solutions (drugs, vaccines, etc.) that act at the physical and physiological level, it loses relevance when it comes to subjective domains such as wellbeing and quality of life. In the latter, the objective researcher mindset must be nurtured from within, at a personal level so it can provide direct one to one guidance to oneself in the subjective aspects that matter the most to oneself.

In the health and wellbeing space, what do I observe? How does this observation help?

We have already discussed the lifestyle choices that confuse us and distract us from the goal. Our vision, personal wellbeing journal, and observer mindset should help us stay on course. In addition, there are deeper and subtle observations that matter much and can give valuable cues for our wellbeing.

If we stay alert, we can detect the reactions of the body and mind to external stimuli very early. This can help us plan and act suitably. For example, trying a new food item and its consequence such as gastritis, or sneezing is a reaction of the body. Even before they manifest as symptoms, the body may react, and many times right at the time we begin to consume them or soon after the first gulp. If we are alert, we can stop right there and avoid the consequences.

Hence, consumption of foods very consciously and slowly is advised. This not only aids digestion and assimilation but also helps to pick up subtler effects much earlier.

Similarly, we are used to a certain quantity of exercises or Yoga that help to remove stiffness and generate strength and fitness. Sometimes, with changing seasons, times, and places, the same quantum may have different effects causing more tiredness or exhaustion in the body or a sense of lethargy in the mind. Staying in tune with the effects and accordingly adjusting the dosage is how the observation helps.

Noting down these effects in your journal will build your personal research and knowledge base, and will prove to be valuable in the long run.

30 IA 4: Be Part of an Inspired Team, Find a Buddy and a Mentor

A *vision, journal,* and *observer mindset,* the three aspects we discussed so far relate to oneself. They help to start the journey and move on. When we tag along with others who are similarly inspired, the journey will be fun and the learning curve is steep. So being part of a like-minded group is highly beneficial.

We are social beings and love to connect and exchange. This drive is stronger in the current times of social media which is giving us plenty of opportunities to share and learn. Sharing a good practice and getting a 'like' is a great incentive and motivation. By sharing, you are inspiring others too.

Forming a peer group in person or on social media, who have a common vision is always a strong force.

We talked about the observation of experiences, effects of food, and exercises on the body and mind. When we share them in our circle, others will benefit from our experience and stay alert. When others share, that makes us more observant too. Especially the practical challenges one faces and the knowledge of how they overcame them are valuable lessons for us. Similarly, our solutions will help others too saving valuable time and energy.

The group can boost our learning and motivation.

These days there is a wealth of wellbeing resources and literature that are available and it is hard to stay updated.

Organizing journal clubs, study groups, and connecting at regular intervals for advancing one's knowledge goes a long way.

Within the group, find a buddy who is more aligned to you.

It could be your life partner, your close friend, or a colleague, one who knows you well. This is someone with whom you can open up and seek feedback. Constructive feedback from someone you trust is valuable and it works just as the objective observer you have.

Lastly, like in any other discipline, you need a guide or a mentor in the health and wellbeing space too.

We hear of many instances of wrong training of fitness or Yoga that leads to undesirable effects. One such experience can become a permanent mental block. Seeking guidance from an expert at the right time is always desirable. This is not just at the time of learning a new lifestyle trait, but also as we move along the journey. Precisely when we hit road-blocks, when body and mind throw up reactions, it is time to connect with the mentor and take help. Their experience on their path will be a valuable practical lesson for us.

So, an inspired team includes you, your circle, your buddy, and your mentor. Together along with your inner resources, they form an invincible strength.

31 IA 5: Strive to Become a Champion

The idea of becoming a wellbeing champion puts us off in the very beginning. It is related to one's confidence, other goals and priorities, work pressures, and many more factors. We often relate to this term from an outsider's perspective.

Nonetheless, it can be purely a personal idea too wherein you are striving to be a champion not to the world out there, but for yourself.

It is similar to the idea of leadership; it has external and internal connotations.

What makes someone a champion? How is a champion different from the others?

While there are many characteristics, a few standout:

- being vision oriented and able to stay committed to the vision,
- being self-motivated and able to do course-corrections,
- be a supporting hand and a source of inspiration to others.

Whether we like to become a champion or not, the first two are important for everyone who aspires to enjoy good health and wellbeing, as we have discussed in the chapters so far. The last one is something that will happen naturally and spontaneously and is a result of the first two. So why not strive to become a champion?

You can be a source of inspiration to others in more than one way.

You can become a trainer yourself or a coach and probably this can be yet another profession too. If not a job, it can simply be another hobby and a part-time, volunteer work too.

There are other ways as well…

You can share your experiences through blogs and articles; you can form your own peer group and facilitate exchange amongst the group members.

You can share a scientific article or a book, share what appeals to you and invite others' insights; you can take a lead in forming study groups, or host a few journal clubs.

In a natural way, you begin to touch others' hearts and will be seen as a useful resource.

If you would like, you may host webinars and give presentations to your circles of friends, colleagues, and relatives. Who knows a book and a TED talk may follow soon, and before you realize, the world would recognize you as a champion. All this can happen in a natural way without the least pressure on one's mind.

To a true champion, only the vision is in sight and the efforts at the moment are all that matters. It's not too complex. Isn't it?

SECTION 4

Lifestyle Change for Common Conditions: *Practical Integrative Approach (PIA) Series*

Note:

For all the conditions in this section, standard treatment protocols exist and continue to be the norm as prescribed by a trained physician. The practices and recommendations from other fields are suggested as part of lifestyle recommendations, to complement mainstay treatments.

In no way, the primary treatment should be discontinued or interrupted. Any additional intervention, including that of the lifestyle change, should be informed to the treating physician.

Similarly, the Ayurveda, Yoga, and Meditation related services should be sought from certified and skilled trainers.

PIA 1: Coronaviruses and Covid-19 Disease

Introduction

Coronaviruses are a group of viruses that affect the respiratory system. Severe Acute Respiratory Syndrome (SARS), Middle East Respiratory Syndrome (MERS), and now, the novel Corona or Covid-19, they all belong to the Corona family.

The disease caused by the most recent (novel) Coronavirus is called Corona Virus Disease (Covid-19). The virus is named as SARS Corona Virus 2 (SARS Cov 2). The first case was reported by China in the city of Wuhan in December 2019.

In a short span of ten months, the virus spread across more than 200 countries, infecting over 33 million people and killing more than 1,000,000 individuals. This rapid transmission is attributed to the human lifestyle as well as the nature of the virus itself (infectivity).

Transmission

Initial transmission in China has been reported as due to animal-human contact (from bats).

Later, person-to-person transmission through direct contact or through droplets (cough, sneeze) from an infected person caused the spread of the disease.

The virus primarily attacks the lining of the respiratory system by binding to the receptors on the cells, called ACE2 (angiotensin converting enzyme 2) receptor.

Clinical Features

Fever, tiredness, and dry cough are common.

Others include sneezing, running nose, sore throat, and loose stools (diarrhoea).

Complicated cases develop pneumonia.

The cases with fever, cough, difficulty in breathing should seek medical help.

80-85% of infected cases experience mild symptoms and will recover. About 15% may develop complications, and 3-5% tend to die.

The complications and deaths are reported mostly in the elderly, those having underlying medical conditions like cardiovascular diseases, diabetes, chronic respiratory disease, cancers, etc.

Current Management Options

Complicated cases will need hospitalization and ventilator support.

Currently, no drug or vaccine is proven and trials are still in progress.

Hence, all suspected cases with a history of Covid symptoms should be tested and managed appropriately.

Quarantine (isolate) the infected case to prevent further transmission.

Identify all contacts of the infected case and test them, quarantine those who test positive.

Closely monitor for symptoms while adopting personal preventive measures.

Prevention Measures

Prevention becomes critical when no drug or vaccine is available. Prevention is important at the individual, family, and societal levels. Hence people, governments, and all stakeholders have to work together.

Watch out for the guidelines of the local government and Public Health Administrators and plan accordingly. Adhere to the following WHO's recommendations for personal prevention:

- *Wash your hands regularly with soap and water, or clean them with alcohol-based hand rub.*
- *Maintain at least a one-meter distance between you and others. Wear a cotton mask that covers your mouth and nose.*
- *Avoid touching your face.*
- *Stay home if you feel unwell.*
- *Refrain from smoking and other activities that weaken the lungs.*
- *Practice physical distancing by avoiding unnecessary travel and staying away from large groups of people.*

Integrative Lifestyle Advise[10]

Strengthen general immunity, prevent respiratory symptoms through the control of *Vata* and *Kapha doshas* that are mainly implicated in the respiratory infections as per the Ayurveda theory:

- *Drink warm water.*
- *Use ginger, pepper, garlic in the foods. Coriander, cumin, and turmeric are helpful.*

---

[10] For specifics related to Ayurveda, Yoga and Meditation, refer to corresponding good to know sections

- *Avoid cold foods, including curds (yogurt), as well as deep fried and processed foods.*
- *Stay indoors: consume freshly prepared, warm food every time.*
- *Avoid exposure to winds directly.*
- *Practice whole body or head oil massage (Abhyanga) at regular intervals. Refer to particular oils for a particular constitution and for a particular season.*
- *In addition, smear few drops of warmed, cooled coconut oil into the nostrils for local immunity.*
- *Cleanse the nasal passage using a 'Neti' pot administering saline or salt water in the mornings.*

Continue the Yoga asanas as per your constitution for general immunity, body flexibility, and vitality. Pranayama exercises are particularly helpful for the lungs and the other body systems:

- *Full Yogic breathing improves the quality of inhalation and exhalation and revitalizes the whole body.*
- *Alternate nostril breathing or Nadi suddi pranayama helps to improve oxygen intake and eliminate carbon dioxide.*
- *Kapalabhati cleanses the respiratory passage, improves the quality of breathing (oxygen and carbon dioxide movement), and improves digestion.*

If your physical condition permits, continue to meditate and follow other supportive practices as recommended by the Heartfulness Institute to stay calm and centered, to relieve you of any stress or anxiety associated with the illness.

Important Dos and Don'ts

Dos	Don'ts
Ensure 100% compliance with standard prevention and treatment guidelines. Stay in touch with your Ayurveda physician for any advice and treatment including the Neti procedure. Learn Yoga asanas and pranayama from a certified and skilled Yoga instructor.	Don't stop or interrupt standard treatment procedures and guidelines. Kapalabhati is best avoided in hypertension, abdominal pain, or cramps. Keep your primary physician informed of all the lifestyle practices you follow.

33 PIA 2: Diabetes Mellitus

Introduction

Diabetes is a chronic medical condition characterized by high glucose (sugar) levels in the blood. The high blood glucose will eventually damage blood vessels, heart, eyes, kidneys, and nerves.

In the normal course, the pancreas secretes insulin which will clear the glucose from the blood into the cells, soon after meal intake. If diabetes is a result of little or no insulin secretion from the pancreas, due to certain pre-conditions (an autoimmune disorder that damages the pancreas), it is referred to as **Type 1 Diabetes**. When seen in children, this is referred as Juvenile Diabetes.

A more common type is **Type 2 Diabetes** (85-95%), which will be the focus of this chapter. Type 2 Diabetes is due to two reasons: 1) reduction in the secretion of insulin; 2) resistance of cells to the action of insulin (insulin resistance). It is commonly seen after 40 years of age and has an association with family history and obesity.

Type 2 Diabetes was previously seen mainly in the developed countries, but recently, it is on a rise in developing countries too due to various factors: social changes, urbanization, dietary changes, reduced physical activity, and unhealthy lifestyles.

WHO estimates that the world has about 422 million diabetics and every year, about 1.6 million deaths are attributed to Diabetes.

Pathophysiology

Glucose levels increase in the blood due to the following processes:

- In the fed state, due to intestinal absorption of the foods consumed.
- In the fasting state, from two sources: 1) breakdown of glycogen in the liver and, 2) formation of new glucose out of amino acids and lactate.

The insulin hormone is responsible for clearing any excess glucose in the blood soon after the meals; the glucose is driven into the cells of the skeletal muscles and fat in the body. Insulin also stops the release of glucose into the blood from other sources: breakdown of glycogen in the liver and formation out of amino acids.

Thus, the insulin hormone plays a critical role in the regulation of glucose homeostasis, with support from other hormones, glucagon (has the opposite effect – stimulates the appearance of glucose in blood), amylin, and incretin (both complement insulin).

In Type 2 Diabetes, there is a resistance to insulin as well as reduced secretion of insulin, amylin, and incretin which lead to higher glucose in the blood, referred to as hyperglycemia.

Diagnosis

Glucose tolerance tests, random blood sugar, post-prandial blood sugar (after a meal), fasting blood sugar (early morning after 12 hours of overnight fasting), Glycosylated hemoglobin (HB1Ac) test (aggregate glucose levels over the last 12 weeks) are common diagnostic methods used.

Point of care tests are available for self-diagnosis and screening, and positive, it is important to see a physician, to confirm the diagnosis.

All Type 2 Diabetes mellitus will go through a prediabetes state when high blood glucose levels are still reversible. It is important to screen for blood sugar at regular intervals, after 40 years of age, especially when any risk factors are predisposing to diabetes. Regular screening helps in early detection and effective management.

Clinical Features

Common symptoms due to high blood glucose are frequent urination (polyuria), drinking of water (polydipsia), eating (polyphagia), and tiredness, etc.

Over time, the high blood glucose damages different systems and results in blurred or loss of vision (retinopathy), nerve tingling and pain (neuropathy), kidney symptoms (nephropathy), cardiovascular symptoms (chest pain, heart attack, etc.).

Foot damage and amputation, skin infections, hearing loss, dementia, and depression are a result of uncontrolled diabetes.

Current Management Options

- The focus of Type 2 Diabetes management is to maintain optimal blood glucose levels, and prevent the occurrence of complications and premature death.
- WHO recommends modification of the following risk factors:
  - o Adopt healthy eating habits

- o   Start physical activity
- o   Stop smoking
- o   Control blood pressure
- o   Control lipids (fats)
- Drugs to lower blood glucose and blood pressure as per the standard treatment guidelines.
- Regular screening of eyes (retinoscopy), kidneys (urine proteins), and feet (foot examination) to monitor and prevent complications.

Prevention of diabetes

- *Maintain healthy body weight and avoid weight gain in adulthood*
- *Increase physical activity and reduce sedentary behaviors*
- *Replace saturated and trans fats with unsaturated fats*
- *Replace refined grains with whole grains*
- *Avoiding smoking and alcohol*

Integrative Lifestyle Advice[11]

As per the Ayurveda school of thought, the root cause is diet and lifestyle disturbance which disturbs an individual's innate constitution (*Prakriti*) and management lies in rectifying the same. Lifestyle disorders are referred to as *Prameha*. Hence, it is advised to:

Understand one's constitution through the examination of pulse and detailed history from an Ayurveda physician.

---

[11] For specifics related to Ayurveda, Yoga and Meditation, refer to corresponding good to know sections

Adopt a lifestyle and food practice that is unique to the individual's constitution. They include:

- Avoid a sedentary lifestyle
- Avoid excessive sleep as well as sleeping during the day
- Fix a time for your meals
- Avoid excess curds/ yogurt/ dairy products
- Avoid processed foods

Complement the lifestyle change with specific herbal and panchakarma treatments to balance the constitution.

Constantly monitor the blood glucose levels while maintaining compliance with the primary treating physician.

Following Yoga asanas have the potential to stimulate the pancreas and increase insulin secretion as well as in improving insulin sensitivity.

Suryanamaskara, Tadasana, Katichakrasana, Sarvangasana, Halasana, Matsyasana, Ushtrasana, Gomukhasana, Ardhamatsyendrasana, Mandukasana, Paschimottanasana, Pawanmuktaasana, Bhujangasana, Shalabhasana, Dhanurasana, Vajrasana, Shavasana

Pranayamas (breathing exercises) improve the quality of breathing, metabolism, and energy.

Kapalabhati, Nadi suddi pranayama, Sitakari, Bhramari, Suryabhedi, Bhastrika

Meditation helps to stay calm and stress-free and indirectly can affect blood glucose levels through the regulation of the autonomic nervous system. Rightly done, it helps to develop discrimination and make the right choices with regards to lifestyle, food practices, and treatment compliance.

Important Dos and Don'ts

Dos	Don'ts
Ensure total compliance with standard prevention and treatment guidelines. Stay in touch with your Ayurveda physician for any advice and treatment for lifestyle in general or diabetes in particular. Learn Yoga asanas and pranayama from a certified and skilled Yoga therapy instructor. Keep your physician informed of the lifestyle changes you are adopting. Monitor the blood glucose levels at regular intervals and accordingly modify the Ayurveda and Yoga regimen.	Never stop treatment or follow up visits with your primary physician who is treating diabetes. Don't make drastic changes in lifestyle, but do it in alignment with your body-mind capacity, while continuing to monitor blood glucose control. Don't delay reporting any side-effects as a result of disease or any lifestyle change. Don't stop taking standard drugs or reduce dosage because you start other practices. Let your treating physician decide the dosage and change based on the improvements.

PIA 3: Hypertension and Cardiovascular Diseases

Introduction

Hypertension refers to a medical condition that shows persistently high levels of blood pressure. If uncontrolled, it will increase the risk of heart, brain, kidney diseases, and premature death. WHO estimates 1.13 billion people as having hypertension in the world.

Cardiovascular diseases (CVDs) are a group of disorders related to the heart and blood vessels and include coronary heart diseases (where blood vessels of the heart are affected), cerebrovascular disease (blood vessels of the brain), peripheral arterial disease (vessels of arms and legs), and rheumatic heart disease (damage to the heart muscle and heart valves due to streptococcal infection).

CVDs are the leading cause of death today contributing to about 18 million deaths worldwide every year. Just two CVDs- heart attack and stroke contribute to 85% of all CVD deaths.

Pathophysiology

Heart attacks are caused when the blood vessels supplying the blood to the heart are blocked due to fat deposition on the inner lining of the vessel walls. Similarly, stroke is caused when blood vessels of the brain are blocked. Strokes can also be due to bleeding from the blood vessel or from a blood clot.

An unhealthy diet, physical inactivity, tobacco, and alcohol are the key behavioral risk factors that lead to high blood pressure, high blood glucose, high lipids, overweight, and obesity, which together predispose one to any of the CVDs.

Diabetes is particularly a strong risk factor. The natural regulation of contraction and dilation of small vessels, a function of the autonomic nervous system is affected in diabetic neuropathy. This results in a poorer exchange of nutrients and metabolic products between the blood and the tissues, giving rise to tissue damage. Also, diabetes results in presence of chronic inflammatory cytokines, free radicals, and hypercoagulability of blood, all that are implicated in heart failure.

Hypertension and CVDs are seen commonly among those above 65 years of age, have a family history and co-existing disease.

Diagnosis and Monitoring

Blood pressure, blood sugar, kidney function tests, lipid profile, eye examination, and other assessments, are advised at regular intervals to monitor for control of hypertension and complications.

Clinical Features

Hypertension may not show any symptoms for a long time. It can manifest as early morning headache, nose bleeds, vision changes, buzzing in the ears, and irregular heart rhythms.

Severe forms may present as nausea, vomiting, confusion, fatigue, muscle tremors, chest pain.

If untreated, hypertension along with other risk factors may lead to chronic chest pain (angina), heart attack, heart failure, and an irregular heart-beat that may lead to sudden death.

Heart attack or stroke can sometimes be the first warning without any clue to the underlying disease.

Heart attack presents as pain or discomfort in the chest, arms, left shoulder, elbow, jaw, or back. This may be accompanied by shortness of breath, vomiting, faint attack, and becoming pale.

A stroke will present commonly as sudden weakness of the face, arm, or leg, mostly on one side of the body. It may be accompanied by numbness of the affected parts, confusion, speech and vision changes, difficulty in walking and understanding, severe headache, fainting, and loss of consciousness.

Current Management Options Including Prevention

Manage the modifiable risk factors:

- Reduce salt intake (to less than 5g daily)
- Eat more fruits and vegetables
- Consume whole grain foods
- Limit saturated fats and eliminate trans fats in the diet
- Reduce weight through regular physical activity
- Avoid the use of tobacco
- Reduce alcohol consumption

If uncontrolled, blood pressure lowering drugs, management of stress, and other underlying medical conditions are required as per the standard treatment guidelines, in addition to the risk factor management.

For heart attack and stroke, prevention of the first episode is the priority; this is also referred to as primary prevention and achieved through control of blood pressure and cholesterol.

Once the CVD is established, preventing further complications is achieved through secondary prevention. Drugs for the prevention of coagulation of blood (aspirin), to lower BP (beta blockers, ACE inhibitors) and cholesterol (statins) are used.

Integrative Lifestyle Advice[12]

Ayurveda explores the role of three *doshas* in the management of hypertension and gives valuable advice on prevention and health promotion, rather than targeting the disease directly:

- Reduce intake of oily, salty, sour, and spicy foods, that can aggravate Pitta dosha that is implicated in Hypertension.
- Reduce weight.
- Specific foods can set right the imbalance of doshas: Barley (Yava), sorghum (Jowar), wheat, green gram (Mudga/ Moong dal), horse gram (Kulatha), moringa (Shigru), Bitter gourd (karela), bottle gourd (Ghia/Lauki), turnip (Shalgam), carrot (Gajar), radish (Muli), Indian gooseberry (Amla), cucumber (Kira), black grapes (Draksha), pomegranate (Anar), apple, pineapple, cold milk, etc.
- Avoid excess butter, ghee, and animal fats.
- Avoid smoking and alcohol consumption.
- Fix sleep and wake-up time. Avoid daytime sleeping.

---

[12] For specifics related to Ayurveda, Yoga and Meditation, refer to corresponding good to know sections

- *Specific herbal and panchakarma treatments will balance the doshas. Shirodhara and Takradhara are advised to manage stress and relax the body and the mind.*
- *Constantly monitor the blood pressure through regular follow-ups with the primary treating physician.*

Yoga aims to regulate blood circulation and normalizes blood pressure through its effects on the autonomic nervous system. Specific Yoga postures can be explored:

Tadasana, Katichakrasana, Konasana, Uttanapadasana, Pavanamuktasana, Vajrasana, Ushtrasana, Shashankasana, Bhujangasana, Gomukhasana, Makarasana, Vakrasana, Shavasana

Pranayama exercises affect the autonomic nervous system, reduce the blood pressure, calm the mind.

Nadi shudhi, Sitali, Sitakari, Sadanta, Bhramari, Ujjayi

Meditation complements other interventions, regulates the parasympathetic nervous system, and slows down heart rate, respiration, and blood pressure. Meditation can also act indirectly through the reduction of stress and anxiety. Refer to Heartfulness Meditation and other supportive practices in the annexure.

Important Dos and Don'ts

Dos	Don'ts
Ensure absolute compliance with standard prevention and treatment guidelines for hypertension and CVD. Stay in touch with your Ayurveda physician for any advice and treatment for lifestyle in general or hypertension in particular. Learn Yoga asanas and pranayama from a certified and skilled Yoga therapy instructor. Keep your physician informed of the lifestyle changes you are adopting. Monitor the blood pressure levels and other CVD-related indicators, at regular intervals and accordingly modify the Ayurveda and Yoga regimen. Do Yoga asanas with awareness and assessment of its effects on your body.	Do not interrupt your treatment or follow-up visits with your primary physician who is treating hypertension or CVD. Do not engage in any Yoga asanas when you have severe CVD. Avoid head-standing (Shirsasana) and hyperventilation. Do not delay reporting of any side-effects to the experts, but seek timely advice. Do not change Ayurveda or Yoga regimen yourself, but seek an expert's help. Don't stop taking standard drugs or reduce dosage because you start other practices. Let your treating physician decide the dosage and change based on the improvements.

35 PIA 4: Mental Health: Depression, Anxiety, and Stress

Introduction

20% of the world's children and adolescents have one or other mental health conditions. Suicide is the second leading cause of death among 15-29 year-olds.

These mental health conditions affect performance at schools and workplaces, and relationships within the family. Just two conditions: depression and anxiety, cost US$ 1 trillion of the global economy every year.

Among the elderly, dementia, depression, and anxiety are common mental health disorders and significantly affect the quality of life of patients as well as care-givers.

Contributing Factors

They result from a complex interaction of the social, psychological, and biological factors. Psychological trauma, work and performance-related stress, bereavement, relationship issues have been implicated in depression.

Depression can lead to stress and dysfunction. Depression can be a result of medical disorders, especially chronic diseases.

Activation of the Hypothalamic Pituitary Adrenocortical (HPA) axis due to excess levels of corticotrophin-releasing hormones in the blood is implicated. HPA axis, in the normal course, is the natural stress response to an external situation; it is short-lived until the time the threat exists and prepares the body to combat stress. During this response, an increase in blood pressure, heart rate, respiration, diversion of blood from the brain to muscles, is observed. A prolonged stimulus will lead to chronic stress resulting in adverse health issues.

Chronic stress can lead to anxiety and depression.

Clinical Features

Chronic stress can result in headaches, high blood pressure, chest pain, palpitations, and loss of sleep

In chronic depression, one notices a depressed mood, loss of interest and enjoyment, reduced energy, and activity. Feelings of guilt, low self-worth, disturbed sleep and appetite, anxiety and poor concentration, decreased sex drive, feelings of helplessness and hopelessness, are also observed.

While mild cases of depression can have some difficulty in carrying on day to day activities, severe cases will not be able to continue their domestic or social activities.

Current Management Options

Everyone experiences symptoms related to depression, anxiety, and stress some time or the other. If they persist for long and affect the quality of life and performance, help has to be sought from counselors and physicians.

Symptoms of depression, anxiety, and stress often coexist.

Counseling and psychotherapy is the first line in mild cases.

Antidepressant medications are reserved for moderate to severe conditions.

Integrative Lifestyle Advice[13]

Ayurveda theory implicates excess of one of the three doshas in depression. The following advice is only to be used as complementary to mainstay treatments. So, the assessment of doshas is important to identify the right etiology of depression.

Vata type depression is associated with fear, anxiety, nervousness, and insomnia.

- Domestic remedies like Dashamoola tea, tea from ashwaganda and brahmi, or tulsi (basil) can help.
- Nose drops of warm sesame oil, massage on the top of the head and soles with sesame will pacify Vata.
- Avoiding loneliness.

Pitta type depression is associated with anger, fear of failure, loss of control, or suicidal thoughts. The following domestic remedies can pacify excess pitta:

- Oil massage in the scalp with coconut or sunflower oil
- Brahmi, Jatamamsi or Shatavari in tea
- Brahmi ghee as nose drops
- Relaxation pose, slow breathing, and Meditation are helpful to calm the body and mind

The Kapha depression presents with mental heaviness, excess sleep, weight gain, drowsiness. The following remedies will help:

- Fasting supported by apple juice reduces heaviness

---

[13] For specifics related to Ayurveda, Yoga, and Meditation, refer to corresponding good to know sections

- Increase exercises
- Ginger tea
- Herbs such as saraswati, punarmava, and chitrak
- Yoga - Sun salutation and breathing exercises (ujjai pranayama) will help

Stress also has similar roots in Vata, Pitta, and Kapha doshas and has to be managed accordingly. In addition to the above, one should perform long deep breathing, oil massage, and Meditation.

Anxiety is associated with fears, insomnia, and is primarily due to aggravation of Vata.

- Tea made of musta and tagar (valerian) is calming
- Full body oil massage, relaxing bath
- Almond milk, Orange juice
- Yoga – relaxation pose (Savasana), slow breathing, left nostril breathing, and Meditation can calm down the system through their effects on the autonomic nervous systems and HPA axis

Generally, the Yoga and pranayama exercises should be chosen after assessing one's constitution. In addition, time and space for contemplation, revisiting the larger picture of life, and planning lifestyle changes is helpful.

These apply in mild to moderate cases, and in addition to the routine treatments. In moderate to severe cases, where many of the above recommendations are not feasible, it is important not to force oneself, but to take the help of a counselor and/or a physician to achieve the optimal state of mind before trying some of the above remedies.

Important Dos and Don'ts

Dos	Don'ts
If any of the clinical symptoms persist for longer periods, consult a physician (psychiatrist) and counselor for assessing the degree of severity and need for medication. Ensure absolute compliance with standard prevention and treatment guidelines. The Ayurveda, Yoga, and Meditation are advised as adjuvant treatments to support the mainstay treatment and not otherwise, and seek help from experts. Keep your physician informed of the lifestyle changes you are adopting.	Do not interrupt your treatment or follow up visits with your primary physician or counselor. Do not change Ayurveda or Yoga regimen, yourself, but seek an expert's help. Do not try Meditation in severe cases.

PIA 5: Cancers

Introduction

Cancer is a group of disorders characterized by a rapid rate of growth of abnormal cells that will invade neighboring and distant parts of the body. This is referred to as metastasis indicating advanced stages of cancer. They can affect any organ or body system.

Cancers are the second leading cause of death, next only to cardiovascular diseases. In 2018, 9.6 million deaths were estimated as due to cancers.

A third of the cancer deaths are due to one of the following risk factors: high body mass index, low physical activity, less intake of fruits and vegetables, smoking, and alcohol.

Causes and Factors Involved

It is not clear as to why some develop and some do not, yet some risk factors are associated with cancers.

The causes range from genetic factors to carcinogens that stimulate the growth of abnormal cells.

- Environmental: Exposure to ultraviolet and ionizing radiation, air pollution.
- Lifestyle: tobacco, food practices.

- Chemical: exposure to asbestos, arsenic, benzene
- Infections: Human Papilloma virus, Herpes, Hepatitis, Helicobacter, etc.
- Pesticides, herbicides, electromagnetic radiation, genetically modified crops, artificial growth hormones are reported though the evidence is not conclusive.

The carcinogen leads to genetic defects and causes cell damage and their proliferation. When the immune system fails to check the growth of the abnormal cells, they continue to proliferate and lead to cancerous states. New blood vessels in the tumors supply nutrition and oxygen and facilitate further expansion.

Clinical Features and Diagnosis

Cancer symptoms vary widely depending on the organ that is involved and the extent of involvement.

General features include rapid weight loss, anemia, fatigue or tiredness, and loss of appetite.

Diagnosis varies by type of cancer: lab tests for blood count and specific tumor markers, biopsy, and imaging tests are done.

Staging of cancers helps to assess the extent and spread of cancers if they have involved other organs and lymph nodes. Tumor grading helps to assess the level of abnormality, and the potential to grow and spread. Jointly, they help to know the severity, and potential for recovery and in planning management.

Current Management Options

Screening and early detection is critical for effective management of the cancers.

Surgery, radiation therapy, and chemotherapy are standard modalities available for cancer treatment.

In advanced cancers, palliative treatment is resorted to, which is focused on improving quality of life, rather than curing cancer.

Prevention

WHO recommends modification or avoidance of the following risk factors as a prevention strategy:

- Tobacco use including cigarettes and smokeless tobacco
- Overweight or obesity
- Unhealthy diet with low fruit and vegetable intake
- Lack of physical activity
- Alcohol use
- Sexually transmitted HPV-infection
- Infection by hepatitis or other carcinogenic infections
- Urban air pollution
- Indoor smoke from household use of solid fuels
- Vaccinate against HPV and hepatitis B virus
- Control of occupational hazards
- Reduce exposure to ultraviolet radiation
- Reduce exposure to ionizing radiation (occupational or medical diagnostic imaging)

Integrative Lifestyle Advice[14]

In Ayurveda, cancer can be the result of either an inflammatory or non-inflammatory process, and the tumor can be minor

---

[14] General prevention based on one's constitution is the mainstay. Refer to Good to Know series for more specific details.

(Granthi) or major (Arbuda). They are linked to aggravated Vata and Kapha doshas. Some are treatable and some aren't and hence, the emphasis is laid on prevention. Lifestyle changes are advised as follows:

- Consume a balanced and healthy diet, with a lot of vegetables and fruits.
- Avoid tobacco and alcohol.
- Specific herbs are indicated for specific types of cancers; they can complement mainstay treatments.

Yoga exercises and breathing techniques are of help to build immunity and vitality, facilitate lymphatic movement, and activation of the autonomic nervous system which have roles in cancer progression.

- Surya Namaskar, Tadasana, Ushtrasana, Vakrasana, Gomukhasana, Bhujangasana, Shalabhasana, Dhanurasana, Simhasana, Shavasana.
- Kapalabhati, Nadishodhana, Ujjai, Shitali, Sitkari, Bhastrika.

Meditation and other integrative health practices are important for not just the clients but also the family members who go through enormous stress and anxiety in the process. Meditation can help navigate the situation smoothly; it can bring about acceptance of the situation, facilitate appropriate decision making in these challenging times, and more importantly can provide inner peace and harmony.

Note:

- Cancer diagnosis results in a lot of stress and panic both in the client and the family members. This gets compounded and confusing when hearing experiences from others of what works and what doesn't. Evidence-based practice is always the mainstay and should be the starting point. Based on how the body responds to the main treatment and in consultation with the treating physician, the management should be planned carefully.

- Integrative approaches have a significant role at all stages of cancer progression. In the initial stages and especially during chemotherapy when the body immunity deteriorates, the integrative approaches can be helpful. The Ayurveda lifestyle and customized dietary recommendations alongside Yoga and Meditation can build immunity and mental resilience from within.

- In the advanced stages when the conventional treatments are not effective, integrative approaches can restore the quality of life through changes in the mental and emotional realms. More so when Ayurveda or Yoga is not possible, simple breathing exercises, relaxation, and Meditations that Heartfulness Institute offers can be very helpful. Hundreds of cancer patients who are supported through Heartfulness practices, over the years, have reported improved calm, peace, and acceptance of the phase. Families too that go through enormous stress during these stages have reported changes in mental and emotional states.

- Cancer treatments result in immunosuppression and complications that can be lethal. Careful watch during chemotherapy is critical. Any additional treatment including the integrative approaches and treatments should not result in complications. The primary physician has to be kept informed at all stages.

Important Dos and Don'ts

Dos	Don'ts
Conventional, evidence based practice is the mainstay. Consult the physician at all stages of the condition.	Do not interrupt your treatment or follow up visits with your primary physician or counselor.
The Ayurveda, Yoga, and Meditation are advised as adjuvant treatments to support the mainstay treatment and seek to help them from experts.	Do not start or modify Ayurveda or Yoga regimen, yourself, but seek expert help.
Keep your physician informed of the lifestyle changes you are adopting and any additional treatment you may be considering as there can be interactions and side-effects.	Don't mechanically force any integrative health lifestyle on to the client, but ensure natural and seamless integration.
At times of stress and anxiety, seek the help of the counselor.	
Keep the client and their interest always in the center, while processing decisions.	
Continue to monitor the progress for any decisions, in consultation with the physician.	

SECTION 5

Annexures: Resources, Tools, and Support

RTS 1: Self-Assessment Tool

*T*his is a self-assessment tool to explore one's constitution. No person is completely a Vata or Pitta or a Kapha, but a combination of the three and one or two may predominate. You may score by ticking those that form your general pattern most of the year, and later, sum it up to understand how the three doshas spread out within your constitution.

Do not forget to get a pulse examination done by an Ayurveda physician for confirmation of your constitution, both Prakriti as well as Vikruti.

Characteristics	VATA	PITTA	KAPHA
Body Frame	❑ Thin	❑ Moderate	❑ Well Built
Body Weight	❑ Low	❑ Moderate	❑ Overweight / Obese
Skin	❑ Dry, Rough, Cool	❑ Soft, Oily, Warm, Fair, Sensitive	❑ Thick, Oily, Cool, Pale Fair
Hair	❑ Dry, Easy to break, Split ends	❑ Soft, oily, early greying, baldness	❑ Thick, oily, wavy, dark, or light.
Teeth	❑ Protruded, big, crooked teeth, gums emaciated	❑ Moderate in size, soft gums, yellowish teeth	❑ Strong & white Teeth
Eyes	❑ Small, dull, dry	❑ Sharp, shiny, penetrating.	❑ Big, attractive, thick eyelashes

Characteristics	VATA	PITTA	KAPHA
Tongue	❑ Cracked, impression of teeth, black-brown spots	❑ Red, yellow coating	❑ White coated
Appetite	❑ Variable (Too hungry or no hunger keeps changing)	❑ Good, Excessive	❑ Slow but steady
Preferred Tastes	❑ Salty, sour, sweet	❑ Sweet, bitter, astringent	❑ Pungent, bitter, astringent
Thirst	❑ Variable	❑ Excessive	❑ Scanty
Bowel	❑ Dry, hard, constipated	❑ Soft, oily, loose	❑ Thick, oily, heavy, slow
Physical Activity	❑ Very Active	❑ Moderate	❑ Lethargic
Mental Activity	❑ Restless, active	❑ Moderate	❑ Dull, Slow
Emotions	❑ Fearful, Insecure, Anxious, Unpredictable,	❑ Aggressive, Intelligent, ❑ Critical, Analytical	❑ Possessive, Greedy, Calm, Composed, Depression, ❑ Attractive personality
Faith /Beliefs	❑ Easily Influenced by others	❑ Passionate, Steady	❑ Slow in trusting others but steady
Memory	❑ Quick to understand, Quick to forget	❑ Sharp	❑ Slow but prolonged
Dreams	❑ Fearful, Flying, Jumping	❑ Fiery, anger, violence war	❑ Water, River, Ocean
Sleep	❑ Light sleeper, disturbed sleep	❑ Light sleeper, Sound sleep	❑ Prolonged Sleeper, Sound sleep
Speech	❑ Fast, Cluttered, Un-organized	❑ Continuous, Organized, Specific	❑ Slow, organized, elongated
Voice	❑ Harsh, Rustic Voice	❑ Husky, Base voice	❑ Melodious, Nectar like Voice
Total Score	❑	❑	❑

38 RTS 2: Personal Wellbeing Journal Tool and Tracke

Based on the changes you want to bring about in your lifestyle, identify the top 3 priorities under different categories for this month. List them in the tool. Implement them and tick against the days of the months when you are able to comply.

My Priorities for this month				
LIFESTYLE MEDICINE	AYURVEDA REMEDIES	YOGA ASANAS & PRANAYAMA	HFN MEDITATION PRACTICES	OTHERS
1. 2. 3.	1. 2. 3.	1. 2. 3.	1. 2. 3.	1. 2. 3.
MONTHLY COMPLIANCE TRACKER				

L1																															
L2																															
L3																															
A1																															
A2																															
A3																															
Y1																															
Y2																															
Y3																															
H1																															
H2																															
H3																															
O1																															
O2																															
O3																															
O4																															
O5																															
O6																															

RTS 3: Heartfulness Practices

Heartfulness Relaxation

Read through these guided suggestions and try them on yourself or read them aloud to help guide others. This practice works best when you turn off your phone and other devices that might distract you. Relaxation can be done at any time and is especially useful before beginning Heartfulness Meditation.

Sit comfortably and close your eyes very softly and very gently.

Begin with your toes. Wiggle your toes. Now feel them relax.

Feel the healing energy of Mother Earth move up into your toes, feet, and ankles. Then up to your knees, relaxing the lower legs.

Feel the healing energy move further up your legs. Relax your thighs.

Now, deeply relax your hips, lower body, and waist.

Relax your back. From your tailbone to your shoulders, feel your entire back relaxing.

Relax your chest and shoulders. Feel your shoulders simply melting away.

Relax your upper arms. Relax each muscle in your forearms, your hands, and right to your fingertips.

Relax your neck muscles. Move your awareness up to your face. Relax your jaw, mouth, nose, eyes, earlobes, facial muscles, forehead... all the way to the top of your head.

Feel your whole body completely relaxed. Scan your system from top to toe, and if there is any part of your body that is still tense, painful, or unwell, feel it being immersed in the healing energy of Mother Earth for a little longer.

When you are ready, move your attention to your heart. Rest there for a little while. Feel immersed in the love and light in your heart.

Remain still and quiet, and slowly become absorbed within.

Remain absorbed for as long as you want, until you feel ready to come out.

Heartfulness Meditation

Choose a place where you can meditate without being distracted, preferably at the same place and time daily. The most ideal time of the day is before sunrise.

Turn off your phone and other devices. Sit with your back upright but not rigid.

Sit comfortably. Gently close your eyes and relax.

If needed, take a couple of minutes to relax your body by doing the Heartfulness Relaxation.

Turn your attention inward and take a moment to observe yourself.

Then, suppose that the Source of the Divine Light is already present within your heart and that it is attracting you from within.

Gently relax into that feeling. If you find your awareness drifting to other thoughts, do not fight them but also do not entertain them. Let them be, while simply reminding yourself that you are meditating on the Source of Divine Light in your heart.

Allow yourself to become more and more absorbed within.

Remain absorbed within this deep silence for as long as you want, until you feel ready to come out of Meditation.

Heartfulness Cleaning

Do the cleaning practice at the end of your day's work, preferably around sunset, and not too close to bedtime. This process will rejuvenate you and purify your system of any accumulated heaviness. There are a few steps to the cleaning process, so in the beginning, it is best to use the following sequence:

Sit in a comfortable position with the intention to remove all the impressions accumulated during the day.

Close your eyes and relax.

Imagine all the complexities and impurities are leaving your entire system.

Let them flow out from your back in the form of smoke, from the area between your tailbone (at the base of your spine) and the top of your head.

Remain alert during the entire process without brooding over the thoughts and feelings that arise. Try to remain a witness to your thoughts.

Gently accelerate this process with confidence and determination.

If your attention drifts and other thoughts come to mind, gently bring your focus back to the cleaning.

As the impressions are leaving from your back, you will start to feel lighter.

Continue this process for twenty to twenty-five minutes.

When you feel light within, you can start the second part of the process.

Feel a current of purity coming from the Source entering your system from the front. This current is flowing into your heart and throughout your system, saturating every particle.

You have now returned to a more balanced state. Every particle of your body is emanating lightness, purity, and simplicity.

Finish with the conviction that the cleaning has been completed effectively.

Heartfulness Prayer

This prayer is offered at bedtime, as a way of connecting to the Source before sleep. This may take around ten to fifteen minutes. It is also offered before Meditation in the morning.

At bedtime, sit comfortably, gently close your eyes, and relax. Silently and slowly repeat the words of the prayer below. Meditate for ten to fifteen minutes over the true meaning, feeling the words resonate in your heart rather than trying to analyze them. Let the meaning surface from within. Try to get lost in it. Go beyond the words and let the feeling come to you.

O' Master! Thou art the real goal of human life.

We are yet but slaves of wishes putting bar to our advancement.

Thou art the only God and Power to bring us up to that stage.

Now silently repeat these words a second time and go even deeper into this feeling. Allow yourself to be absorbed in the feeling beyond the words. Allow yourself to melt in this prayerfully meditative state as you go to sleep.

In the morning, reconnect yourself by silently offering this prayer once before you start the Heartfulness Meditation.

Health, Wellbeing, and Quality of Life: *Changing Paradigm*

1. Ferranti P. The United Nations Sustainable Development Goals. In: Encyclopedia of Food Security and Sustainability. 2018.
2. World Health Organization. SDG Health and Health-Related Targets. World Health Statistics. 2016.
3. Roser, M., Ortiz-Ospina, E., & Ritchie, H. (2020). Life Expectancy. Retrieved 23 August 2020, from https://ourworldindata.org/life-expectancy
4. Disease burden and mortality estimates. (2020). Retrieved 23 August 2020, from https://www.who.int/healthinfo/global_burden_disease/estimates/en/index1.html
5. Megari K. Quality of life in chronic disease patients. Heal Psychol Res. 2013;
6. Crimmins EM. Lifespan and healthspan: Past, present, and promise. Gerontologist. 2015;
7. Varni JW, Limbers CA, Burwinkle TM. Impaired health-related quality of life in children and adolescents with chronic conditions: A comparative analysis of 10 disease clusters and 33 disease categories/severities utilizing the PedsQLTM 4.0 Generic Core Scales. Health Qual Life Outcomes. 2007;
8. Vanhoutte B. The Multidimensional Structure of Subjective Well-Being In Later Life. J Popul Ageing. 2014;
9. Vanhoutte B, Nazroo J. Cognitive, affective and eudemonic well-being in later life: Measurement equivalence over gender and life stage. Sociol Res Online. 2014;

10. Meiselman HL. Quality of life, well-being and wellness: Measuring subjective health for foods and other products. Food Qual Prefer. 2016;

11. 8 Dimensions of Wellness. (2020). Retrieved 23 August 2020, from https://umwellness.wordpress.com/8-dimensions-of-wellness/

12. WHO. WHOQOL Measuring Quality of Life. Psychol Med. 1998;

13. Noah C Peeri, Nistha Shrestha, Md Siddikur Rahman, Rafdzah Zaki, Zhengqi Tan, Saana Bibi, Mahdi Baghbanzadeh, Nasrin Aghamohammadi, Wenyi Zhang, Ubydul Haque, The SARS, MERS, and novel coronavirus (COVID-19) epidemics, the newest and biggest global health threats: what lessons have we learned?, *International Journal of Epidemiology*, dyaa033

14. Conor Stewart. Lifestyle changes made dye to coronavirus in Great Britain. March 2020

Lifestyle Change and Challenges: *Unanswered Questions*

15. H Nawaz, C M. Via, A Ali, L D Rosenberger. Project ASPIRE: Incorporating Integrative Medicine into Residency Training. Am J Prev Med. 2015 Nov; 49(5 0 3): S296–S301

16. Integrative Medicine Training for Family Physicians. (2020). Retrieved 23 August 2020, from https://www.stfm.org/ publicationsresearch/publications/educationcolumns/2011/ june/

17. Saylee Deshmukh, Mahesh Vyas, Hitesh Vyas, Dwivedi R R (2015). Concept of Lifestyle in Ayurveda Classics. Global J Res. Med. Plants & Indigen. Med., Volume 4(2): 30–37

18. Bombardieri D, Easthope G. Convergence between orthodox and alternative medicine: A theoretical elaboration and empirical test. Health. 2000;4:479–94

19. Debra Campbell and Kathleen Moore (2004) Yoga as a Preventative and Treatment for Depression, Anxiety, and Stress. International Journal of Yoga Therapy: 2004, Vol. 14, No. 1, pp. 53-58.

20. Jayaram Thimmapuram et al (2020) Heartfulness meditation improves sleep in chronic insomnia, Journal of Community Hospital Internal Medicine Perspectives, 10:1, 10-15,

21. Hardcastle et al (2015). Motivating the unmotivated: how can health behavior be changed in those unwilling to change?. Frontiers in psychology, 6, 835.

22. Kähkönen, et al (2015). Motivation is a crucial factor for adherence to a healthy lifestyle among people with coronary heart disease after percutaneous coronary intervention. Journal of advanced nursing. 71. 10.1111/jan.12708.

23. Ross C. L. (2009). Integral healthcare: the benefits and challenges of integrating complementary and alternative medicine with a conventional healthcare practice. Integrative medicine insights, 4, 13–20. https://doi.org/10.4137/imi.s2239

24. Angie Drakulich. Challenges faced when implementing an integrative care model. Meeting Highlights. AIPM Global Pain Clinician Summit 2018

25. Wang C (2014). Challenges for the Future of Complementary and Integrative Care. Health Care Current Reviews 2: e102. doi: 10.4172/2375-4275.1000e102

26. Huang J, Yu H, Marin E, Brock S, Carden D, Davis T. Physicians' weight loss counseling in two public hospital primary care clinics. Acad Med. 2004;79(2): 156-161

Integrative Health and Wellbeing: *An Introduction*

27. National Center for Complementary and Integrative Health. Complementary, Alternative, or Integrative Health: What 's In a Name? National Center for Complementary and Alternative Medicine. 2015.

28. Clarke TC, Black LI, Stussman BJ, Barnes PM, Nahin RL. Trends in the use of complementary health approaches among adults: United States, 2002-2012. Natl Health Stat Report. 2015;

29. Bishop FL, Yardley L, Lewith GT. A systematic review of beliefs involved in the use of complementary and alternative medicine. J Health Psychol. 2007;

30. What is Integrative Healthcare? - Duke Integrative Medicine. (2020). Retrieved 23 August 2020, from https://dukeintegrativemedicine.org/leadership-program/what-is-integrative-healthcare/

31. Cohen, M. Challenges and Future Directions for Integrative Medicine in Clinical Practice. Evid-Based-Integrative-Med 2, 117–122 (2005).

32. Medicine, U. (2020). Why does Integrative Medicine Matter? - Explore Integrative Medicine. Retrieved 23 August 2020, from https://exploreim.ucla.edu/video/why-integrative-medicine-matters/

33. (2020). Retrieved 23 August 2020, from https://www.cihw.in/well-being-centers

Lifestyle Medicine Series

34. Eilat-Adar S, Xu J, Zephier E, O'Leary V, Howard BV, Resnick HE. Adherence to dietary recommendations for saturated fat, fiber, and sodium is low in American Indians and other US adults with diabetes. J Nutr. 2008;138(9):1699- 1704

35. Lianov L, Johnson M. Physician Competencies for Prescribing Lifestyle Medicine. JAMA. 2010;304(2):202–203. doi:10.1001/jama.2010.903

36. Krishnamurthy Jayanna, N. Swaroop, Arin Kar, et al. Designing a comprehensive Non- Communicable Diseases (NCD) programme for hypertension and diabetes at primary health care level: evidence and experience from urban Karnataka, South India. BMC Public Health (2019) 19:409

37. Stafford RS, Farhat JH,Misra B, Schoenfeld DA. National patterns of physician activities related to obesity management. Arch Fam Med. 2000;9(7):631-638

38. Calfas KJ, Long BJ, Sallis JF, Wooten WJ, Pratt M, Patrick K. A controlled trial of physician counseling to promote the adoption of physical activity. Prev Med. 1996;25(3):225-233

39. Partnership for Prevention Preventive Care: A National Profile on Use, Disparities, and Health Benefits. Washington, DC: Partnership for Prevention; August 2007.

40. Loef, M., Walach, H., 2012. The combined effects of healthy lifestyle behaviours on all-cause mortality: a systematic review and meta-analysis. Prev. Med. 55, 163–170.

41. Uddin, R.; Lee, E.Y.; Khan, S.R.; Tremblay, M.S.; Khan, A. Clustering of lifestyle risk factors for non-communicable diseases in 304,779 adolescents from 89 countries: A global perspective. Prev. Med. 2019, 131, 105955

42. Egger, G, Binns, A & Rossner, S 2011, *Lifestyle medicine: managing diseases of lifestyle in the 21st century*, 2nd edn, McGraw-Hill, North Ryde, NSW

43. Egger G, Binns A, Rossner S. Lifestyle medicine. Sydney: McGraw-Hill Australia, 2008

Nutrition: *Energy, Metabolism and Healthy Diet*

44. Kim E. Barrett, Susan M. Barman, Scott Boitano, Heddwen Brooks. Ganong's Review of Medical Physiology. New Delhi: McGraw-Hill Education (India), 2016

45. Morton GJ, Schwartz MW. Int J Obes Relat Metab Disord. 2001 Dec; 25 Suppl 5():S56-62

46. Keesey RE, Powley TL. Appetite. 2008 Nov; 51(3):442-5

47. Healthy diet. (2020). Retrieved 23 August 2020, from https://www.who.int/news-room/fact-sheets/detail/healthy-diet

48. Johnstone AM, Murison SD, Duncan JS, Rance KA, Speakman JR. Factors influencing variation in basal metabolic rate include fat-free mass, fat mass, age, and circulating thyroxine but not sex, circulating leptin, or triiodothyronine. Am J Clin Nutr. 2005 Nov; 82(5):941-8

49. Diet, nutrition and the prevention of chronic diseases: report of a Joint WHO/FAO Expert Consultation. WHO Technical Report Series, No. 916. Geneva: World Health Organization; 2003.

50. Guidelines: Saturated fatty acid and *trans*-fatty acid intake for adults and children. Geneva: World Health Organization; 2018 (Draft issued for public consultation in May 2018).

51. Guideline: Sugars intake for adults and children. Geneva: World Health Organization; 2015.

52. Guideline: Sodium intake for adults and children. Geneva: World Health Organization; 2012.

Sleep: *Circadian rhythm, Biological Clock and Healthy Sleep*

53. The Nobel Prize in Physiology or Medicine 2017. NobelPrize. org. Nobel Media AB 2020. Tue. 19 May 2020

54. M. Garaulet, P. Gómez-Abellán, J. J. Alburquerque-Béjar, Y. C. Lee, J. M. Ordovás, F. A. Scheer. Timing of food intake predicts weight loss effectiveness. Int. J. Obes. 37, 604–611 (2013).

55. S Panda. Circadian physiology of metabolism. SCIENCE25 NOV 2016 : 1008-1015

56. Irwin, M., Opp, M. Sleep Health: Reciprocal Regulation of Sleep and Innate Immunity. Neuropsychopharmacol 42, 129–155 (2017)

57. Garaulet, M., Gómez-Abellán, P., Alburquerque-Béjar, J. et al. Timing of food intake predicts weight loss effectiveness. Int J Obes 37, 604–611 (2013)

58. Irwin, M., Opp, M. Sleep Health: Reciprocal Regulation of Sleep and Innate Immunity. Neuropsychopharmacol 42, 129–155 (2017)

59. Naresh M. Punjabi, et al. Sleep-Disordered Breathing, Glucose Intolerance, and Insulin Resistance: The Sleep Heart Health Study, *American Journal of Epidemiology*, Volume 160, Issue 6, 15 September 2004, Pages 521–530

60. J.J. PILCHER et al. Sleep quality versus sleep quantity: relationships between sleep and measures of health, well-being and sleepiness in college students. Journal of Psychosomatic Research, Vol. 42, No. 6, pp. 583 596. 1997

61. Capuccio et al. Sleep Duration and Obesity. SLEEP, Vol. 31, No. 5, 2008

62. C. A. Czeisler and J. J. Gooley. Sleep and Circadian Rhythms in Humans. Cold Spring Harbor Symposia on Quantitative Biology, Volume LXXII. © 2007 C

63. Dashti HS, Scheer FA, Jacques PF, et al. Short sleep duration and dietary intake: epidemiologic evidence, mechanisms, and health implications. Adv Nutr 2015;6:648–59.

64. Vioque, J., Torres, A. & Quiles, J. Time spent watching television, sleep duration and obesity in adults living in Valencia, Spain. Int J Obes 24, 1683–1688 (2000)

65. Burgess, Helen J, and Thomas A Molina. "Home Lighting Before Usual Bedtime Impacts Circadian Timing: A Field Study." Photochemistry and photobiology. 90.3 (2014): 723–726. Web

66. Hale L, Kirschen GW, LeBourgeois MK, et al. Youth Screen Media Habits and Sleep: Sleep-Friendly Screen Behavior Recommendations for Clinicians, Educators, and Parents. Child Adolesc Psychiatr Clin N Am. 2018;27(2):229-245.

67. Maw SS, Haga C. Effect of a 2-hour interval between dinner and bedtime on glycated haemoglobin levels in middle-aged and elderly Japanese people: a longitudinal analysis of 3-year health check-up data. BMJ Nutrition, Prevention & Health 2019

68. Khalsa, S.B.S. Treatment of Chronic Insomnia with Yoga: A Preliminary Study with Sleep–Wake Diaries. Appl Psychophysiol Biofeedback 29, 269–278 (2004)

69. Jayaram Thimmapuram, Deborah Yommer, Luminita Tudor, Theodore Bell, Cristian Dumitrescu & Robert Davis (2020) Heartfulness meditation improves sleep in chronic insomnia, Journal of Community Hospital Internal Medicine Perspectives, 10:1, 10-15,

70. Vera Abeln, Jens Kleinert, Heiko K. Strüder & Stefan Schneider (2014) Brainwave entrainment for better sleep and post-sleep state of young elite soccer players – A pilot study, European Journal of Sport Science, 14:5, 393-402

71. Wang, Chun-Fang, Ying-Li Sun, and Hong-Xin Zang. "Music Therapy Improves Sleep Quality in Acute and Chronic Sleep Disorders: A Meta-Analysis of 10 Randomized Studies." International journal of nursing studies. 51.1 (2014): 51–62. Web.

Physical Activity: *Physiology, Benefits, and Recommendations*

72. Physical activity. (2020). Retrieved 23 August 2020, from https://www.who.int/news-room/fact-sheets/detail/physical-activity

73. Patel PN, Zwibel H. Physiology, Exercise. [Updated 2019 May 5]. In: StatPearls [Internet]. Treasure Island (FL): StatPearls Publishing; 2020

74. Abdin S, Lavallée JF, Faulkner J, Husted M. A systematic review of the effectiveness of physical activity interventions in adults with breast cancer by physical activity type and mode of participation. Psychooncology. 2019 Jul;28(7):1381-1393

75. Carbone S, Billingsley HE, Rodriguez-Miguelez P, Kirkman DL, Garten R, Franco RL, Lee DC, Lavie CJ. Lean Mass Abnormalities in Heart Failure: The Role of Sarcopenia, Sarcopenic Obesity, and Cachexia. Curr Probl Cardiol. 2019 Mar 28;:100417

76. Ibeneme SC, Omeje C, Myezwa H, Ezeofor SN, Anieto EM, Irem F, Nnamani AO, Ezenwankwo FE, Ibeneme GC. Effects of physical exercises on inflammatory biomarkers and cardiopulmonary function in patients living with HIV: a systematic review with meta-analysis. BMC Infect. Dis. 2019 Apr 29;19(1):359

77. Kramer SF, Hung SH, Brodtmann A. The Impact of Physical Activity Before and After Stroke on Stroke Risk and Recovery: a Narrative Review. Curr Neurol Neurosci Rep. 2019 Apr 22;19(6):28

78. Liu N, Gou WH, Wang J, Chen DD, Sun WJ, Guo PP, Zhang XH, Zhang W. Effects of exercise on pregnant women's quality of life: A systematic review. Eur. J. Obstet. Gynecol. Reprod. Biol. 2019 Nov;242:170-177

79. Publishing, H. (2020). The 4 most important types of exercise - Harvard Health. Retrieved 23 August 2020, from https://www.health.harvard.edu/exercise-and-fitness/the-4-most-important-types-of-exercise

80. Tobacco and Alcohol: *Effects, Physiology and Healthy Recommendations*

81. Tobacco. (2020). Retrieved 23 August 2020, from https://www.who.int/news-room/fact-sheets/detail/tobacco

82. Alcohol. (2020). Retrieved 23 August 2020, from https://www.who.int/news-room/fact-sheets/detail/alcohol

83. Innes, E. (2013, Mar 13). Men smoke to have fun, but for stressed-out women, it's all about preserving inner calm. *Mail Online*

84. Milner D. The physiological effects of smoking on the respiratory system. *Nurs Times*. 2004;100(24):56-59.

85. Audrain-McGovern J, Benowitz NL. Cigarette smoking, nicotine, and body weight. *Clin Pharmacol Ther*. 2011;90(1):164-168. doi:10.1038/clpt.2011.105

86. Benowitz NL. Nicotine addiction. *N Engl J Med*. 2010;362(24):2295-2303. doi:10.1056/NEJMra0809890

87. Clapp, P., Wackernah, R., & Minnick, M. (2014). Alcohol use disorder: pathophysiology, effects, and pharmacologic options for treatment. *Substance Abuse And Rehabilitation*, 1. doi: 10.2147/sar.s37907

88. George, O. (2015, Apr 14). TSRI Scientists Find that Nicotine Use Increases Compulsive Alcohol Consumption. *The Scripps Research Institute (TSRI)*

89. Aminde LN, Takah NF, Zapata-Diomedi B, Veerman JL. Primary and secondary prevention interventions for cardiovascular disease in low-income and middle-income countries: a systematic review of economic evaluations. *Cost Eff Resour Alloc*. 2018;16:22. Published 2018 Jun 14. doi:10.1186/s12962-018-0108-9

Stress and Immunity: *Effects, Physiology, and Healthy Behaviors*

90. Le Fevre, Mark, Jonathan Matheny, and Gregory S Kolt. "Eustress, Distress, and Interpretation in Occupational Stress." *Journal of managerial psychology*. 18.7 (2003): 726–744. Web

91. Ströhle A. The neuroendocrinology of stress and the pathophysiology and therapy of depression and anxiety. Nervenarzt. 2003 Mar;74(3):279-91

92. Benson, H., & Allen, R. (1980). How much stress is too much? *Harvard Business Review, 58*, 86–92.

93. Types of Stressors (Eustress vs. Distress). (2020). Retrieved 23 August 2020, from https://www.mentalhelp.net/articles/types-of-stressors-eustress-vs-distress/

94. McGonigal, K. (2013). *How to make stress your friend*. Ted Global, Edinburgh, Scotland, 6, 13.

95. Thimmapuram J, Pargament R, Sibliss K, Grim R, Risques R, Toorens E. Effect of heartfulness meditation on burnout, emotional wellness, and telomere length in health care professionals. J Community Hosp Intern Med Perspect. 2017

96. Debra Campbell and Kathleen Moore (2004) Yoga as a Preventative and Treatment for Depression, Anxiety, and Stress. International Journal of Yoga Therapy: 2004, Vol. 14, No. 1, pp. 53-58.

97. ter Horst R, Jaeger M, Smeekens S et al. Host and Environmental Factor Influencing Individual Human Cytokine Responses. 2016, Cell167, 1111–1124

98. Segerstrom SC, Miller GE. Psychological stress and the human immune system: a meta-analytic study of 30 years of inquiry. Psychol Bull. 2004;130:601–630
Steptoe A, Hamer M, Chida Y. The effects of acute psychological stress on circulating inflammatory factors in humans: a review and meta-analysis. Brain Behav Immun. 2007;21:901–912

99. Gouin JP, Glaser R, Malarkey WB, Beversdorf D, Kiecolt-Glaser J. Chronic stress, daily stressors, and circulating inflammatory markers. Health Psychol. 2012;31:264–268.

100. Morey, J. N., Boggero, I. A., Scott, A. B., & Segerstrom, S. C. (2015). Current Directions in Stress and Human Immune Function. Current opinion in psychology, 5, 13–17. https://doi.org/10.1016/j.copsyc.2015.03.007

Ayurveda Series

101. Nayak J. Ayurveda research: Ontological challenges. J Ayurveda Integr Med 2012;3:17-20

102. Singh: Exploring issues in the development of Ayurvedic research methodology. Journal of Ayurveda & Integrative Medicine | April 2010 | Vol 1 | Issue 2

103. Chandola H M. Lifestyle disorders: Ayurveda with lots of potential for prevention. Year : 2012 | Volume: 33 | Issue Number: 3 | Page: 327-327

104. Saylee Deshmukh, Mahesh Vyas, Hitesh Vyas, Dwivedi R R (2015). Concept of Lifestyle in Ayurveda Classics. Global J Res. Med. Plants & Indigen. Med., Volume 4(2): 30–37

105. Bombardieri D, Easthope G. Convergence between orthodox and alternative medicine: A theoretical elaboration and empirical test. Health. 2000;4:479–94

106. Furst DE, Venkatraman MM, McGann M, Manohar PR, Booth-LaForce C, Sarin R, et al. Double-blind, randomized, controlled, pilot study comparing classic Ayurvedic medicine, methotrexate, and their combination in rheumatoid arthritis. J Clin Rheumatol. 2011;17:185–92

107. Hari Sharma, H.M. Chandola. Ayurvedic Concept of Obesity, Metabolic Syndrome, and Diabetes Mellitus. The Journal of Alternative and Complementary Medicine. Vol 17, No 6, 2011, pp. 549–552

108. Maanasi Menon, Akhilesh Shukla. Understanding Hypertension in the light of Ayurveda. Journal of Ayurveda and Integrative Medicine 9 (2018) 302e307

109. Vasant Lad. The Complementary Book of Ayurvedic Home Remedies. London. 2006.

110. Sivananda Yoga Vedanta Centre. Practical Ayurveda. Great Britain. 2018.

111. David Frawley. Ayurvedic Healing: Comprehensive guide. Wisconsin.2000

112. David Frawley and Subhash Ranade. Ayurveda Nature's Medicine. Delhi. 2011

Yoga Series

113. Kamlesh D Patel. The Profound Beauty of Yoga. Heartfulness Collector's Edition. December 2018

114. Tiffany Field. Yoga clinical research review. Complementary Therapies in Clinical Practice Volume 17, Issue 1, February 2011, Pages 1-8

115. Marshall Hagins, Rebecca States, Terry Selfe, Kim Innes. Effectiveness of Yoga for Hypertension: Systematic Review and Meta-Analysis. Volume 2013, Article ID 649836. Evidence-Based Complementary and Alternative Medicine

116. Debra Campbell and Kathleen Moore (2004) Yoga as a Preventative and Treatment for Depression, Anxiety, and Stress. International Journal of Yoga Therapy: 2004, Vol. 14, No. 1, pp. 53-58.

117. Maheshkumar Kuppusamy, Dilara Kamaldeen, Ravishankar Pitani, et al. Effects of yoga breathing practice on heart rate variability in healthy adolescents: a randomized controlled trial, Integrative Medicine Research, 10.1016/j.imr.2020.01.006, (2020)

118. M. Satyapriya, H.R. Nagendra, R. Nagarathna, V. Padmalatha. Effect of integrated yoga on stress and heart rate variability in pregnant women. Int J Gynaecol Obstet, 104 (2009), pp. 218-222

119. Karen Pilkington, Graham Kirkwood, Hagen Rampes, Janet Richardson. Yoga for depression: The research evidence. Journal of Affective Disorders Volume 89, Issues 1–3, December 2005, Pages 13-24

120. Tolahunase, Madhuri R. et al. 'Yoga- and Meditation-based Lifestyle Intervention Increases Neuroplasticity and Reduces Severity of Major Depressive Disorder: A Randomized Controlled Trial'. 1 Jan. 2018: 423 – 442.

121. Kamlesh D Patel. Yogic Psychology. Heartfulness Collectors' edition. December 2019

122. WHAT IS HEALTH ACCORDING TO... YOGA? — SYNERGIES JOURNAL. (2020). Retrieved 23 August 2020, from http://www.synergies-journal.com/wholesomeness/2014/10/6/what-is-health-according-to-yoga

Meditation (Heartfulness) Series

123. Meditation. (2020). Retrieved 23 August 2020, from https://en.wikipedia.org/wiki/Meditation

124. Reibel DK, Greeson JM, Brainard GC, Rosenzweig S. Mindfulness-based stress reduction and health-related quality of life in a heterogeneous patient population. Gen Hosp Psychiatry. 2001;

125. Ospina MB, Bond K, Karkhaneh M, Tjosvold L, Vandermeer B, Liang Y, et al. Meditation practices for health: state of the research. Evid Rep Technol Assess (Full Rep). 2007;

126. Horowitz S. Health Benefits of Meditation: What the Newest Research Shows. Altern Complement Ther. 2010;

127. Mansky PJ, Wallerstedt DB. Complementary medicine in palliative care and cancer symptom management. Cancer Journal. 2006.

128. Thimmapuram J, Pargament R, Sibliss K, Grim R, Risques R, Toorens E. Effect of heartfulness meditation on burnout, emotional wellness, and telomere length in health care professionals. J Community Hosp Intern Med Perspect. 2017;

129. Arya NK, Singh K, Malik A, Mehrotra R. Effect of Heartfulness cleaning and meditation on heart rate variability. Indian Heart J. 2018;

130. Fortney L, Taylor M. Meditation in Medical Practice: A Review of the Evidence and Practice. Primary Care - Clinics in Office Practice. 2010.

131. Jayaram Thimmapuram, Deborah Yommer, Luminita Tudor, Theodore Bell, Cristian Dumitrescu & Robert Davis (2020) Heartfulness meditation improves sleep in chronic insomnia, Journal of Community Hospital Internal Medicine Perspectives, 10:1, 10-15,

132. Potter PJ, Frisch N. Holistic Assessment and Care: Presence in the Process. Nursing Clinics of North America. 2007;

133. Victorson, D., Kentor, M., Maletich, C., Lawton, R. C., Kaufman, V. H., Borrero, M., ... Berkowitz, C. (2015). Mindfulness Meditation to Promote Wellness and Manage Chronic Disease: A Systematic Review and Meta-Analysis of Mindfulness-Based Randomized Controlled Trials Relevant to Lifestyle Medicine. American Journal of Lifestyle Medicine, 9(3), 185–211.

134. Silvani A, Calandra-Buonaura G, Dampney RAL, Cortelli P. 2016 Brain–heart interactions: physiology and clinical implications.Phil. Trans. R. Soc. A 374: 20150181.

135. Complete Works of Ram Chandra. Volume 1. Spiritual Hierarchy Publication Trust, India. 2009.

136. Daaji. Heartfulness Collector's Edition. Issue 12. 2017

137. Patel, K. *Designing destiny.*

138. Patel, K. (1900). *Heartfulness Way*. Reveal Press.

139. Bhuvanesh S Sylapan, Ajay Kumar Nair, Krishnamurthy Jayanna, et al., Meditation, Well-Being and Cognition in Heartfulness Meditators – A Pilot Study. Consciousness and Cognition 86 (2020) 103032

Fasting and Silence

140. Cabo Rafael, Mattson, Mark P. Effects of Intermittent Fasting on Health, Aging, and Disease. *New England Journal of Medicine*, 2541-2551. 381.2019.

141. Elizabeth F. Sutton, Robbie Beyl, Kate S. Early, William T. Cefalu, Eric Ravussin, Courtney M. Peterson, Early Time-Restricted Feeding Improves Insulin Sensitivity, Blood Pressure, and Oxidative Stress Even without Weight Loss in Men with Prediabetes, Cell Metabolism, Volume 27, Issue 6, 2018, Pages 1212-1221.e3,

142. Nuria Martinez-Lopez, Elena Tarabra, Miriam Toledo, et al. System-wide Benefits of Intermeal Fasting by Autophagy, Cell Metabolism, Volume 26, Issue 6, 2017, Pages 856-871

143. https://psychcentral.com/blog/the-hidden-benefits-of-silence/

144. Bernardi L, Porta C, Sleight P. Cardiovascular, cerebrovascular, and respiratory changes induced by different types of music in musicians and non-musicians: the importance of silence. *Heart*. 2006;92(4):445-452. doi:10.1136/hrt.2005.064600

145. Kirste, Imke & Nicola, Zeina & Kronenberg, Golo & Walker, Tara & Liu, Robert & Kempermann, Gerd. (2013). Is silence golden? Effects of auditory stimuli and their absence on adult hippocampal neurogenesis. Brain structure & function.

Coronaviruses and Covid 19 disease

146. H A Rothan, S N Byrareddy. The epidemiology and pathogenesis of coronavirus disease (COVID-19) outbreak. Journal of Autoimmunity 109 (2020) 102433

147. Coronavirus. (2020). Retrieved 23 August 2020, from https://www.who.int/health-topics/coronavirus

148. Is Rinsing Your Sinuses With Neti Pots Safe?. (2020). Retrieved 23 August 2020, from https://www.fda.gov/consumers/consumer-updates/rinsing-your-sinuses-neti-pots-safe

149. Rastogi S, Pandey DN, Singh RH, COVID-19 Pandemic: A pragmatic plan for Ayurveda Intervention, Journal of Ayurveda and Integrative Medicine

Diabetes Mellitus

150. Diabetes. (2020). Retrieved 23 August 2020, from https://www.who.int/news-room/fact-sheets/detail/diabetes
151. International Diabetes Federation. Diabetes Atlas. 2003
152. Krishnamurthy Jayanna, N. Swaroop, Arin Kar, et al. Designing a comprehensive Non- Communicable Diseases (NCD) program for hypertension and diabetes at primary health care level: evidence and experience from urban Karnataka, South India. BMC Public Health (2019) 19:409
153. S L Aronoff, K Berkowitz, B Shreiner, L Want. Glucose Metabolism and Regulation: Beyond Insulin and Glucagon. Diabetes Spectrum Volume 17, Number 3, 2004
154. Schulze MB1, Hu FB. Primary prevention of diabetes: what can be done and how much can be prevented? Annu Rev Public Health. 2005;26:445-67.
155. Hari Sharma, H.M. Chandola. Ayurvedic Concept of Obesity, Metabolic Syndrome, and Diabetes Mellitus. The Journal of Alternative and Complementary Medicine. Vol 17, No 6, 2011, pp. 549–552

Hypertension and Cardiovascular diseases

156. Cardiovascular diseases (CVDs). (2020). Retrieved 23 August 2020, from https://www.who.int/news-room/fact-sheets/detail/cardiovascular-diseases-(cvds)
157. Betsy B. Dokken. The Pathophysiology of Cardiovascular Disease and Diabetes: Beyond Blood Pressure and Lipids. Diabetes Spectrum Volume 21, Number 3, 2008
158. Maanasi Menon, Akhilesh Shukla. Understanding Hypertension in the light of Ayurveda. Journal of Ayurveda and Integrative Medicine 9 (2018) 302e307

159. Vasant Lad. The Complementary Book of Ayurvedic Home Remedies. London. 2006.

160. Marshall Hagins, Rebecca States, Terry Selfe, Kim Innes. Effectiveness of Yoga for Hypertension: Systematic Review and Meta-Analysis. Volume 2013, Article ID 649836. Evidence-Based Complementary and Alternative Medicine

161. Horowitz S. Health Benefits of Meditation: What the Newest Research Shows. Altern Complement Ther. 2010

162. Government of India: Integration of Ayush (Ayurveda) with national program for prevention and control of cancer, diabetes, cardiovascular diseases, and stroke. New Delhi. 2019

Mental Health

163. Mental health. (2020). Retrieved 23 August 2020, from https://www.who.int/westernpacific/health-topics/mental-health

164. Depression. (2020). Retrieved 23 August 2020, from https://www.who.int/news-room/fact-sheets/detail/depression

165. Ströhle A. The neuroendocrinology of stress and the pathophysiology and therapy of depression and anxiety. Nervenarzt. 2003 Mar;74(3):279-91

166. Vasant Lad. The Complementary Book of Ayurvedic Home Remedies. London. 2006.

167. Sundquist, J., Lilja, Å, Palmér, K., Memon, A., Wang, X., Johansson, L., & Sundquist, K. (2015). Mindfulness group therapy in primary care patients with depression, anxiety, and stress and adjustment disorders: Randomised controlled trial. British Journal of Psychiatry, 206(2), 128-135.

168. Debra Campbell and Kathleen Moore (2004) Yoga as a Preventative and Treatment for Depression, Anxiety, and Stress. International Journal of Yoga Therapy: 2004, Vol. 14, No. 1, pp. 53-58.

169. Thimmapuram J, Pargament R, Sibliss K, Grim R, Risques R, Toorens E. Effect of heartfulness meditation on burnout, emotional wellness, and telomere length in health care professionals. J Community Hosp Intern Med Perspect. 2017

Cancers

170. Cancer. (2020). Retrieved 23 August 2020, from https://www.who.int/news-room/fact-sheets/detail/cancer
171. Strohmeyer D. Pathophysiology of tumor angiogenesis and its relevance in renal cell cancer. Anticancer Res. 1999 Mar-Apr;19(2C):1557-61
172. The Genetics of Cancer. (2020). Retrieved 23 August 2020, from https://www.cancer.gov/about-cancer/causes-prevention/genetics
173. S Singh, S K Singh, and N K Singh. Cancer in Ayurveda. International Journal of Basic and Applied Medical Sciences ISSN: 2277-2103
174. Government of India: Integration of Ayush (Ayurveda) with national program for prevention and control of cancer, diabetes, cardiovascular diseases, and stroke. New Delhi. 2019

Future Directions for Integrative Health

175. National Center for Complementary and Integrative Health. Complementary, Alternative, or Integrative Health: What's In a Name? National Center for Complementary and Alternative Medicine. 2015
176. Clarke TC, Black LI, Stussman BJ, Barnes PM, Nahin RL. Trends in the use of complementary health approaches among adults: the United States, 2002-2012. Natl Health Stat Report. 2015
177. Nayak J. Ayurveda research: Ontological challenges. J Ayurveda Integr Med 2012;3:17-20
178. Singh: Exploring issues in the development of Ayurvedic research methodology. Journal of Ayurveda & Integrative Medicine | April 2010 | Vol 1 | Issue 2

ABOUT THE AUTHOR

Dr. Krishnamurthy Jayanna is the founder and director of the Center for Integrative Health and Wellbeing. By training, he is a community health physician and has been active in the public health and development space for close to two decades. His program and research interests revolve around the quality of care, the quality of life, and wellbeing.

Krishnamurthy has been a volunteer at Heartfulness Institute, a Meditation practitioner for nearly 25 years, and a trainer for close to 15 years. He is also an advocate of Yoga. His keen interest and passion in exploring the benefits of Meditation, Yoga, and Natural living, for community health and wellbeing, led him to establish the Center.

In the past, he was part of the global health team of the University of Manitoba, Canada, and was extensively involved in its public health projects across India and Africa. He currently works as Professor and Associate Dean: Research at Ramaiah University of Applied Sciences, where he teaches public health and supports multidisciplinary research. He continues to hold an adjunct faculty position with the Department of Community Health Sciences, University of Manitoba. He is also on the senior advisory team of Karnataka Health Promotion Trust and India Health Action Trust that implements large scale public health projects in India.

He completed M.B.B.S from JSS Medical College, Mysore, India; MD in Community Medicine from Bangalore Medical College, India; received training in research methods at WHO, Geneva, and also holds a post-doctoral research fellowship from Canada.